The Digital Wellness Revolution: Maximizing Internet-based Health Platforms

Jennifer

Copyright © [2023]

Title: The Digital Wellness Revolution: Maximizing Internet-based Health Platforms
Author's: Jennifer

All rights reserved. No part of this publication may be reproduced, stored in a retrieval system, or transmitted in any form or by any means, electronic, mechanical, photocopying, recording, or otherwise, without the prior written permission of the publisher or author, except in the case of brief quotations embodied in critical reviews and certain other non-commercial uses permitted by copyright law.

This book was printed and published by [Publisher's: **Jennifer**] in [2023]

ISBN:

TABLE OF CONTENT

Chapter 1: Introduction to Internet-based Health Platforms　　08

The Rise of Digital Health

Defining Internet-based Health Platforms

Benefits of Internet-based Health Platforms

Chapter 2: The Importance of Digital Wellness　　14

Understanding Digital Wellness

The Impact of Digital Technology on Health

The Need for Balance in the Digital Age

Chapter 3: Exploring Internet-based Health Platforms 20

Types of Internet-based Health Platforms

Fitness and Nutrition Apps

Telemedicine Platforms

Mental Health and Meditation Apps

Personal Health Trackers

How Internet-based Health Platforms Work

Data Collection and Analysis

User Interface and Experience

Feedback and Progress Tracking

Chapter 4: Maximizing Health and Wellness with Digital Platforms   38

Setting Health Goals

Identifying Your Health Priorities

Setting Realistic and Measurable Goals

Leveraging Digital Tools for Exercise and Nutrition

Finding the Right Fitness App or Program

Tracking and Analyzing Nutritional Intake

Utilizing Telemedicine for Remote Care

Accessing Virtual Doctor Consultations

Remote Monitoring and Chronic Disease Management

Promoting Mental Health and Well-being Online

Exploring Meditation and Mindfulness Apps

Connecting with Online Support Communities

Chapter 5: Overcoming Challenges and Ensuring Digital Wellbeing   62

Privacy and Security Concerns

Protecting Personal Health Information

Evaluating Platform Security Measures

Addressing Digital Addiction

Recognizing the Signs of Digital Addiction

Implementing Healthy Digital Habits

Bridging the Digital Divide

Accessibility and Inclusivity in Internet-based Health Platforms

Overcoming Barriers to Adoption

Chapter 6: The Future of Internet-based Health Platforms　　　87

Innovations and Advancements

Artificial Intelligence in Health Platforms

Virtual Reality and Augmented Reality Applications

Ethical Considerations in Digital Health

Data Privacy and Consent

Ensuring Ethical Use of AI and Personalization

The Potential Impact on Healthcare Systems

Integrating Internet-based Health Platforms into Traditional Healthcare

Redefining Healthcare Delivery Models

Chapter 7: Conclusion　　　138

Recap of Key Takeaways

Embracing the Digital Wellness Revolution

Empowering Individuals through Internet-based Health Platforms

Chapter 1: Introduction to Internet-based Health Platforms

The Rise of Digital Health

In today's fast-paced, technology-driven world, it should come as no surprise that the healthcare industry is also experiencing a digital revolution. With the widespread adoption of the internet, digital health has emerged as a powerful force, transforming the way we approach healthcare and empowering individuals to take charge of their own well-being. This subchapter delves into the rise of digital health and explores the myriad benefits it offers to everyone, particularly those connected to the internet.

Digital health refers to the use of internet-based platforms, applications, and technologies to improve health outcomes, enhance communication between patients and healthcare providers, and empower individuals to actively manage their health. The advent of digital health has ushered in a new era of healthcare, characterized by increased access, convenience, and personalized care.

One of the significant advantages of digital health is the accessibility it provides. Through internet-based health platforms, individuals can access a vast array of health information, resources, and tools anytime, anywhere. Whether it's searching for symptoms, learning about a specific condition, or tracking one's fitness goals, the internet has become a treasure trove of health-related knowledge and support.

Moreover, digital health has revolutionized the doctor-patient relationship. With telemedicine, individuals can now consult with healthcare professionals remotely, eliminating the need for in-person visits and long waiting times. This not only saves time and money but also allows patients to receive medical advice and treatment from the comfort of their homes. Additionally, digital health platforms enable seamless communication between patients and healthcare providers, facilitating the exchange of medical records, test results, and treatment plans.

For those connected to the internet, digital health also offers unique opportunities for self-care and personal health management. From wearable fitness trackers to mobile applications that monitor vital signs, individuals can now track their health metrics in real-time, promoting proactive health management and early detection of potential issues. Furthermore, internet-based platforms provide avenues for mental health support, online communities, and virtual coaching, fostering a holistic approach to wellness.

In conclusion, the rise of digital health has transformed the healthcare landscape, offering immense benefits to everyone connected to the internet. From increased accessibility to personalized care and proactive health management, internet-based health platforms have opened up a world of possibilities. As the digital wellness revolution continues to unfold, it is crucial for individuals to embrace these innovative tools and harness their potential for a healthier and happier life.

Defining Internet-based Health Platforms

In today's digital age, the internet has revolutionized various aspects of our lives, including the way we approach healthcare and wellness. Internet-based health platforms have emerged as powerful tools that bridge the gap between individuals and healthcare providers, offering convenience, accessibility, and a wealth of information at our fingertips. This subchapter aims to define and explore the concept of internet-based health platforms, shedding light on their immense potential for revolutionizing the way we manage our health.

Internet-based health platforms, also known as digital health platforms or eHealth platforms, refer to online platforms and applications that provide health-related services, information, and support through the internet. These platforms encompass a wide spectrum of resources, ranging from mobile apps and websites to wearable devices and telemedicine services. The overarching goal of internet-based health platforms is to empower individuals to take control of their health and well-being by leveraging the digital landscape.

One of the key advantages of internet-based health platforms is their accessibility. With a simple internet connection, individuals can access a plethora of health resources and services from the comfort of their homes. Whether it's accessing medical information, monitoring vital signs, booking appointments with healthcare providers, or connecting with support communities, these platforms offer a convenient and time-efficient way to manage one's health.

Moreover, internet-based health platforms are not limited by geographical boundaries, making quality healthcare more accessible to individuals in remote areas or those with mobility limitations. Through telemedicine services, patients can consult with healthcare professionals via video calls, eliminating the need for physical visits to clinics or hospitals.

Additionally, these platforms enable individuals to actively participate in their healthcare journey. With features like health tracking, personalized recommendations, and educational resources, internet-based health platforms empower users to make informed decisions about their lifestyle, diet, exercise, and overall well-being. By fostering a sense of ownership and accountability, these platforms contribute to the promotion of preventive care and proactive health management.

However, it is important to note that internet-based health platforms are not a replacement for traditional healthcare systems or professional medical advice. They should be seen as complementary tools that enhance the overall healthcare experience. It is crucial for individuals to consult with healthcare professionals for accurate diagnoses, treatment plans, and expert guidance.

In conclusion, internet-based health platforms have revolutionized the way we access and manage healthcare. They offer convenience, accessibility, and empowerment by providing a wide range of health resources and services online. However, it is essential for individuals to understand the limitations of these platforms and seek professional medical advice when necessary. The digital wellness revolution is here, and internet-based health platforms are at the forefront, shaping the future of healthcare for everyone.

Benefits of Internet-based Health Platforms

In today's digital age, the internet has revolutionized various aspects of our lives, including the way we manage our health and well-being. Internet-based health platforms have emerged as powerful tools that enable individuals to take charge of their health and make informed decisions. Whether you are a tech-savvy individual or someone who has just ventured into the online world, these platforms provide numerous benefits for people from all walks of life.

One of the key advantages of internet-based health platforms is the ease of accessibility. With just a few clicks, you can access a wealth of information about various health conditions, medications, treatment options, and preventive measures. This accessibility empowers individuals to become active participants in their healthcare journey, fostering a sense of control and autonomy.

Moreover, internet-based health platforms offer a vast array of resources that cater to different needs and preferences. For instance, if you prefer visual aids, you can find informative videos and infographics explaining complex medical concepts. If you are an auditory learner, there are podcasts and audio recordings available at your fingertips. Additionally, these platforms often offer personalized health tracking tools, allowing individuals to monitor their progress and make data-driven decisions.

Another significant benefit of internet-based health platforms is the ability to connect with healthcare professionals and seek expert advice remotely. This virtual consultation feature not only saves time and eliminates the need for physical visits, but it also enables individuals to access healthcare services from the comfort of their own homes. This is particularly beneficial for those living in remote areas or individuals with mobility issues.

Furthermore, internet-based health platforms foster a sense of community and support. Through online forums, social media groups, and virtual support networks, individuals can connect with others facing similar health challenges. This sense of belonging and shared experiences can alleviate feelings of isolation and provide emotional support.

In conclusion, the benefits of internet-based health platforms are far-reaching and cater to everyone, regardless of their familiarity with the internet. These platforms provide easy accessibility to health information, personalized resources, remote consultations, and a sense of community. By embracing the digital wellness revolution, individuals can take control of their health, make informed decisions, and embark on a journey towards a healthier and happier life.

Chapter 2: The Importance of Digital Wellness

Understanding Digital Wellness

In today's digital age, the internet has become an integral part of our lives. It has revolutionized the way we communicate, work, shop, and access information. However, as our dependence on the internet grows, so does the need to prioritize our digital well-being.

Digital wellness refers to the conscious and intentional use of technology to enhance our overall well-being. It encompasses various aspects, including our physical, mental, and emotional health, as well as our social interactions. Understanding digital wellness is crucial for everyone, regardless of their age or occupation, as we are all connected to the internet in some way or another.

One of the key components of digital wellness is maintaining a healthy balance between our online and offline lives. It means being aware of the amount of time we spend online and ensuring that it does not negatively impact our daily routines, relationships, or overall well-being. It also involves setting boundaries and practicing mindful technology use.

Another aspect of digital wellness is protecting our personal information and online privacy. With the increasing threat of cybercrime and data breaches, it is essential to be proactive in safeguarding our digital identities. This can be done by using strong and unique passwords, being cautious while sharing personal information online, and regularly updating privacy settings on social media platforms.

Furthermore, digital wellness includes managing our digital distractions. The internet is filled with endless sources of information and entertainment that can easily divert our attention and affect our productivity. By practicing techniques such as time-blocking, setting device-free zones, and using productivity apps, we can regain control over our online activities and focus on what truly matters.

Additionally, digital wellness encompasses nurturing our mental and emotional well-being in the digital realm. It involves being mindful of our online interactions and cultivating a positive digital footprint. This includes promoting kindness, empathy, and respect in our online interactions, as well as being aware of the potential negative impacts of cyberbullying and online harassment.

In conclusion, understanding digital wellness is paramount in today's internet-driven world. By prioritizing our digital well-being, we can harness the numerous benefits of the internet while mitigating its potential risks. It is essential for everyone to develop healthy habits, set boundaries, protect their privacy, manage distractions, and foster positive online experiences. By doing so, we can maximize the potential of internet-based health platforms and ensure a harmonious integration of technology into our lives.

The Impact of Digital Technology on Health

In today's digital era, the impact of technology on our lives is undeniable. The internet, in particular, has revolutionized the way we access and share information, connect with others, and even manage our health. This subchapter explores the profound influence of digital technology on our well-being and the ways in which the internet has become a powerful tool for improving health outcomes.

Internet-based health platforms have transformed the way we approach healthcare. With just a few clicks, patients can now access a wealth of medical information, connect with healthcare professionals, and even receive virtual consultations. This convenience has made healthcare more accessible and efficient, especially for those in remote areas or with limited mobility. Additionally, patients can now easily schedule appointments, access their medical records, and order prescriptions online, saving valuable time and reducing administrative burdens.

The internet has also empowered individuals to take charge of their own health. Health-tracking apps and wearables allow us to monitor our fitness levels, sleep patterns, and even vital signs. By collecting and analyzing this data, we can gain valuable insights into our overall well-being and make informed decisions to improve our health. Furthermore, online support communities provide a platform for individuals to share experiences, seek advice, and find solace in others facing similar health challenges.

However, it is important to acknowledge the potential downsides of this digital revolution. The ease of access to health information on the internet has led to an overwhelming amount of unverified and misleading content. This can result in individuals self-diagnosing or self-medicating without proper guidance from healthcare professionals. It is crucial to encourage digital literacy and promote reliable sources of information to ensure that individuals make informed decisions about their health.

Moreover, the increased use of digital technology has raised concerns about privacy and data security. As we entrust our personal health information to online platforms, it is essential that robust security measures are in place to protect sensitive data from breaches or misuse. Striking the right balance between convenience and privacy is a challenge that must be addressed to ensure the trust and engagement of individuals in internet-based health platforms.

In conclusion, the impact of digital technology on health is profound and far-reaching. The internet has transformed healthcare, making it more accessible, efficient, and empowering for individuals. Internet-based health platforms have revolutionized the way we access information, connect with healthcare professionals, and monitor our well-being. However, it is crucial to remain vigilant about the potential pitfalls, such as misinformation and data security concerns. By harnessing the power of digital technology while addressing these challenges, we can maximize the benefits and revolutionize the future of healthcare for everyone.

The Need for Balance in the Digital Age

In today's fast-paced and interconnected world, the internet has become an integral part of our daily lives. We rely on it for communication, information, entertainment, and even healthcare. The internet has revolutionized the way we access and manage our health, providing us with a myriad of internet-based health platforms that cater to our diverse needs. However, amidst the convenience and benefits offered by these platforms, there is an urgent need for balance in the digital age.

The internet has undoubtedly brought numerous advantages, especially in the field of healthcare. With just a few clicks, we can now access medical information, connect with healthcare professionals, and even monitor our own health through wearable devices. Internet-based health platforms have made it easier for us to take control of our well-being and make informed decisions about our health.

However, this convenience comes at a cost. The constant exposure to screens and the addictive nature of the internet can have detrimental effects on our physical, mental, and emotional well-being. Excessive use of digital devices has been linked to various health issues, including eye strain, sleep disturbances, and sedentary lifestyles. Moreover, the constant bombardment of information and the pressure to always be connected can lead to stress, anxiety, and a sense of being overwhelmed.

To maintain a healthy and balanced lifestyle in the digital age, it is crucial to set boundaries and establish a conscious relationship with technology. This means finding ways to limit screen time, engage in physical activities, and prioritize face-to-face interactions. It also means being mindful of the quality and reliability of the digital content we consume and being critical of the information we find online.

Finding balance also involves taking regular breaks from the digital world. Unplugging from the internet and engaging in activities that promote relaxation and self-care are essential for our overall well-being. This could include practicing mindfulness, spending time in nature, pursuing hobbies, or simply enjoying moments of solitude.

In conclusion, while internet-based health platforms have revolutionized the way we manage our health, it is crucial to find a balance in the digital age. By setting boundaries, being mindful of our digital consumption, and taking regular breaks, we can ensure that technology enhances rather than hinders our well-being. The internet should be seen as a tool that empowers us to make informed decisions about our health, rather than a source of stress and addiction. Let us embrace the digital wellness revolution while maintaining a healthy balance in our lives.

Chapter 3: Exploring Internet-based Health Platforms

Types of Internet-based Health Platforms

In today's digital era, the internet has become an invaluable tool for accessing health-related information, resources, and services. Internet-based health platforms have revolutionized the way we manage our well-being and have opened up a world of possibilities for individuals seeking to improve their health and quality of life. This subchapter explores the various types of internet-based health platforms that have emerged and how they can benefit everyone in the online community.

1. Health Information Websites: These platforms provide a vast array of health-related information, covering a wide range of topics such as symptoms, disease management, nutrition, and exercise. Health information websites are an excellent resource for individuals seeking to educate themselves on various health conditions, treatment options, and preventive measures.

2. Telemedicine Platforms: Telemedicine platforms enable patients to consult with healthcare professionals remotely. Through video conferencing or phone calls, individuals can receive medical advice, diagnoses, and even prescriptions without the need for an in-person visit. This type of platform is particularly beneficial for those with limited access to healthcare facilities or living in remote areas.

3. Fitness and Wellness Apps: Fitness and wellness apps have gained immense popularity in recent years. These platforms offer personalized workout routines, nutrition tracking, mindfulness exercises, and sleep tracking features. They provide a convenient way

for individuals to stay fit and maintain a healthy lifestyle without the need for expensive gym memberships or personal trainers.

4. Online Support Communities: Internet-based health platforms also facilitate the formation of online support communities. These communities bring together individuals who share similar health concerns, providing a space for them to connect, share experiences, and offer support to one another. Online support communities can be particularly valuable for individuals living with chronic illnesses or rare conditions.

5. Wearable Devices and Health Trackers: With the advancement of technology, wearable devices and health trackers have become increasingly popular. These devices can monitor various health parameters, such as heart rate, sleep patterns, steps taken, and calories burned. They provide individuals with real-time feedback on their health status and can serve as motivation to adopt healthier habits.

In conclusion, the internet has paved the way for a digital wellness revolution, offering a wide range of internet-based health platforms to cater to the diverse needs of individuals. Whether you are seeking information, medical advice, fitness guidance, emotional support, or health tracking tools, internet-based health platforms have something to offer everyone. Embracing these platforms can empower individuals to take charge of their health and well-being, leading to a more fulfilling and healthy life in the digital age.

Fitness and Nutrition Apps

In today's digital era, where the internet has seamlessly integrated into our lives, it has also revolutionized the way we approach fitness and nutrition. With the rise of smartphones and the widespread availability of internet access, a new wave of fitness and nutrition apps has emerged, empowering individuals to take control of their health and well-being like never before.

Fitness apps have become an essential tool for people looking to lead a healthier lifestyle. These apps offer a wide range of features, including personalized workout plans, step counters, calorie trackers, and even virtual personal trainers. Whether you are a beginner or an experienced fitness enthusiast, these apps cater to all levels of expertise, helping you achieve your fitness goals with ease and efficiency. The convenience of having a personal trainer at your fingertips, guiding you through workouts and tracking your progress, is unparalleled.

Nutrition apps, on the other hand, have become indispensable for those seeking to maintain a balanced and healthy diet. These apps provide valuable insights into the nutritional content of various foods and beverages, enabling users to make informed choices about what they consume. Additionally, many nutrition apps offer meal planning and recipe suggestions based on individual dietary preferences and restrictions. With just a few taps on your smartphone, you can create a customized meal plan tailored to your unique needs and goals.

One of the significant advantages of fitness and nutrition apps is their ability to connect with other internet-based health platforms. Most apps seamlessly integrate with fitness trackers, smartwatches, and even social media platforms, allowing users to share their progress, compete with friends, and gain motivation from a supportive online community. These connections foster a sense of accountability and camaraderie, enhancing the overall experience and encouraging users to stay committed to their fitness and nutrition goals.

For internet users of all ages and backgrounds, these fitness and nutrition apps are a gateway to a healthier lifestyle. They provide an accessible and convenient means of taking charge of one's well-being, regardless of time constraints or geographical limitations. Whether you are a busy professional, a stay-at-home parent, or a fitness enthusiast, these apps offer the flexibility and versatility to fit seamlessly into your daily routine.

In conclusion, the advent of fitness and nutrition apps has revolutionized the way we approach health and wellness. With their user-friendly interfaces, personalized features, and integration with other internet-based health platforms, these apps have opened up a world of possibilities for individuals seeking to lead healthier lives. Embrace the digital wellness revolution and harness the power of fitness and nutrition apps to maximize your overall well-being.

Telemedicine Platforms

In today's digital era, the internet has revolutionized various aspects of our lives, and one area that has greatly benefitted from this technological advancement is healthcare. Telemedicine platforms, also known as telehealth platforms, have emerged as a game-changer by leveraging the power of the internet to provide healthcare services remotely. By breaking the barriers of time and distance, these platforms have made quality healthcare more accessible and convenient for everyone.

Telemedicine platforms enable individuals to consult with healthcare professionals through video calls, phone calls, or online messaging. These platforms are not only convenient for patients who cannot visit a physical clinic due to various reasons, but they also prove to be highly efficient for doctors and medical practitioners. With telemedicine, doctors can diagnose and treat patients without the need for in-person visits, reducing waiting times and increasing patient satisfaction.

The internet plays a crucial role in telemedicine platforms, as it serves as the communication medium between patients and healthcare providers. With a stable internet connection, individuals can access a wide range of healthcare services, including primary care, specialty consultations, mental health counseling, and even prescription refills. The internet also allows for the secure transfer of medical records and test results, ensuring that doctors have access to all the necessary information to provide accurate diagnoses and personalized treatment plans.

One of the key advantages of telemedicine platforms is their ability to reach individuals in remote or underserved areas. In regions where access to healthcare facilities is limited, telemedicine bridges the gap by connecting patients with doctors from anywhere in the world. This not only improves healthcare outcomes but also reduces the burden on physical clinics and hospitals.

Moreover, telemedicine platforms have proven to be particularly beneficial during times of crisis, such as the COVID-19 pandemic. With social distancing measures in place, telemedicine became an essential tool for healthcare providers to continue delivering care while minimizing the risk of virus transmission. It allowed patients to receive medical advice and treatment without leaving the safety of their homes.

In conclusion, telemedicine platforms have revolutionized the way healthcare is delivered by harnessing the power of the internet. With these platforms, individuals can access quality healthcare services conveniently, regardless of their geographical location. Through telemedicine, the internet has become a vital tool in bridging the gap between patients and doctors, ensuring that everyone can receive the care they need. As the digital wellness revolution continues, telemedicine platforms will play an increasingly important role in shaping the future of healthcare.

Mental Health and Meditation Apps

In today's fast-paced digital world, where our lives are increasingly intertwined with the internet, it's essential to prioritize our mental well-being. The constant influx of information, social media pressures, and daily stressors can take a toll on our mental health. However, thanks to technological advancements, we now have access to a wide array of tools and resources that can support our mental well-being. One such powerful tool is meditation apps.

Meditation is an age-old practice that has been scientifically proven to reduce stress, anxiety, and depression. It involves focusing one's attention and eliminating the stream of thoughts that often clutter our minds. In recent years, meditation apps have gained immense popularity among people looking for convenient and accessible ways to incorporate mindfulness into their daily routines.

These apps, readily available on the internet, offer a range of guided meditations, breathing exercises, and calming music to help users achieve a state of mental tranquility. They provide personalized experiences tailored to different needs, whether it's stress reduction, improved sleep, or enhanced focus and concentration. The beauty of these apps lies in their ability to bring meditation right to our fingertips, making it accessible anytime, anywhere.

For beginners, meditation apps offer introductory programs that teach the basics of mindfulness and guide users through their initial meditation journeys. These programs are designed to gradually increase the duration and intensity of meditation sessions, allowing users to develop a sustainable practice over time. Additionally, many apps provide reminders and progress tracking features to help users stay consistent and motivated.

Internet-based meditation apps are not only beneficial for individuals but also offer immense value for mental health professionals. Therapists can recommend these apps to their clients as a supplementary tool to support their therapy sessions. Many apps allow users to track their mood, set goals, and even connect with a community of like-minded individuals, fostering a sense of belonging and support.

As with any digital platform, it is crucial to be mindful of the potential downsides of excessive screen time. It is recommended to strike a balance between using meditation apps and engaging in offline activities that promote well-being, such as spending time in nature, practicing yoga, or engaging in face-to-face social interactions.

In conclusion, the internet has revolutionized the way we approach mental health. Meditation apps have emerged as a powerful tool to support our well-being in this digital era. By incorporating these apps into our daily routines, we can harness the benefits of mindfulness and cultivate mental resilience in the face of life's challenges.

Personal Health Trackers

In today's fast-paced digital world, where technology has become an integral part of our lives, it is no surprise that the internet has also revolutionized the way we approach our health and well-being. Personal health trackers have emerged as a powerful tool in this digital wellness revolution, empowering individuals to take control of their own health and make informed decisions.

Personal health trackers, also known as fitness trackers or wearables, are portable devices that monitor and track various aspects of our health and fitness. These devices come in various forms, such as smartwatches, fitness bands, and even smart clothing. They are equipped with sensors that collect data on metrics like heart rate, sleep patterns, steps taken, calories burned, and more.

The internet plays a crucial role in personal health trackers. By connecting these devices to internet-based health platforms, users can access a wealth of information and insights about their health. These platforms provide a centralized hub where users can view and analyze their data, set health goals, track progress, and even share information with healthcare professionals.

One of the key benefits of personal health trackers is their ability to provide real-time feedback. With continuous monitoring, users can gain immediate insights into their health and make adjustments accordingly. For example, if a fitness tracker detects a high heart rate during exercise, it can alert the user to slow down and avoid overexertion.

Internet-based health platforms also offer personalized recommendations and suggestions based on the data collected. These platforms utilize advanced algorithms and artificial intelligence to analyze the data and provide tailored insights. Users can receive personalized workout plans, nutrition advice, and even reminders to stay hydrated or take breaks.

The integration of personal health trackers with the internet has also opened up opportunities for social connectivity and motivation. Many platforms allow users to connect with friends, join challenges, and share their achievements. This social aspect creates a sense of accountability and encourages individuals to stay committed to their health goals.

However, it is important to exercise caution and ensure the privacy and security of personal health data. Users must choose reputable platforms that prioritize data protection and adhere to strict privacy policies.

In conclusion, personal health trackers have become an essential component of the digital wellness revolution. By harnessing the power of the internet, these devices empower individuals to actively monitor and manage their health. With real-time feedback, personalized recommendations, and social connectivity, personal health trackers are revolutionizing the way we approach our well-being in the digital age.

How Internet-based Health Platforms Work

In today's digital age, the internet has revolutionized the way we obtain information and connect with others. This is especially true when it comes to health and wellness. Internet-based health platforms have emerged as powerful tools that enable individuals to take control of their well-being, access healthcare services, and make informed decisions about their health. This chapter will explore how these platforms work and the benefits they offer to everyone in the internet niche.

Internet-based health platforms serve as virtual hubs where individuals can access a wide range of health-related resources and services. These platforms typically offer a variety of features, including online consultations with healthcare professionals, personalized health assessments, access to medical records, and educational materials on various health topics. Users can conveniently access these platforms from the comfort of their own homes, using their computers or mobile devices.

One of the primary functions of internet-based health platforms is to connect individuals with healthcare professionals through online consultations. This allows individuals to seek medical advice and receive diagnoses without the need for physical visits to a clinic or hospital. Through secure video calls or messaging systems, individuals can discuss their symptoms, receive treatment recommendations, and even obtain prescriptions when necessary. This not only saves time and money but also provides access to healthcare services for those who may have difficulty accessing traditional healthcare facilities.

Additionally, these platforms often provide personalized health assessments based on user input and data analysis. By answering a series of questions or inputting relevant information such as age, gender, and lifestyle habits, individuals can receive tailored recommendations for improving their health. This may include suggestions for exercise routines, dietary changes, or preventive measures based on their specific needs.

Internet-based health platforms also enable individuals to access their medical records electronically. This eliminates the need for physical paperwork and allows for easy and secure sharing of information between healthcare providers. Users can view their test results, medication history, and treatment plans, empowering them to actively participate in their own healthcare decision-making process.

Furthermore, these platforms serve as educational resources, offering a wealth of information on various health topics. Users can access articles, videos, and interactive tools to learn about different conditions, treatment options, and preventive measures. This empowers individuals to make informed decisions about their health and take proactive steps towards wellness.

In conclusion, internet-based health platforms have transformed the way we approach healthcare. By leveraging the power of the internet, these platforms provide convenient access to healthcare services, personalized health assessments, electronic medical records, and educational resources. Whether you are seeking medical advice, managing a chronic condition, or simply interested in living a healthier lifestyle, internet-based health platforms offer a wealth of benefits for everyone in the internet niche.

Data Collection and Analysis

In this digital age, the internet has become an integral part of our daily lives. With its vast array of health platforms and resources, it has revolutionized the way we access and manage our well-being. However, with this convenience comes the responsibility of understanding how data collection and analysis play a crucial role in shaping the future of digital wellness.

Data collection is the process of gathering information from various sources, such as online surveys, wearable devices, and health apps. This data holds immense potential to provide valuable insights into our health patterns, behaviors, and overall well-being. By collecting data, we can gain a deeper understanding of our bodies, identify potential health risks, and make informed decisions about our lifestyles.

The internet serves as a vast repository of health-related data, making it an invaluable resource for researchers, healthcare professionals, and individuals. Through the collection of data, we can identify trends and patterns that can aid in the development of personalized health interventions and treatments. Moreover, it enables us to track and monitor our progress towards achieving wellness goals, ultimately empowering us to take control of our own health.

However, data collection is just the beginning. The real power lies in the analysis and interpretation of this data. Through advanced analytics techniques, we can extract meaningful insights and uncover hidden correlations that were previously unknown. This analysis can help us understand the impact of our lifestyle choices on our health, identify factors that contribute to certain conditions, and even predict potential health outcomes.

With the increasing availability of internet-based health platforms, the potential for data collection and analysis has grown exponentially. From wearable fitness trackers to smartphone apps that monitor sleep patterns, the internet offers a plethora of tools to gather data about our health. However, it is important to remember that with this convenience comes the need for privacy and security. Safeguarding our personal health data should be a top priority to ensure it is not misused or accessed by unauthorized individuals.

In conclusion, data collection and analysis are vital components of the digital wellness revolution. The internet provides a wealth of information that can empower individuals to make informed decisions about their health. By harnessing the power of data, we can unlock new insights, understand our bodies better, and take proactive steps towards achieving optimal well-being. However, it is crucial to ensure the security and privacy of our personal health data to maintain trust and confidence in the digital health ecosystem.

User Interface and Experience

In today's digital era, the internet has become an integral part of our lives, offering a multitude of health platforms that empower individuals to take charge of their well-being. However, the success and effectiveness of these internet-based health platforms heavily rely on an often overlooked but crucial aspect: user interface and experience.

The user interface (UI) of a health platform encompasses the design, layout, and presentation of information, while user experience (UX) refers to the overall interaction between the user and the platform. Together, UI and UX play a pivotal role in determining whether individuals will engage with the platform, find it helpful, and ultimately achieve their health goals.

For internet users, a well-designed and intuitive UI is paramount. The interface should be visually appealing, with clear navigation and logical organization of information. By presenting information in a structured and accessible manner, users can easily find what they need, whether it's tracking their fitness progress, monitoring their calorie intake, or accessing educational resources on mental health.

Moreover, a seamless and enjoyable UX is crucial to keep users engaged and motivated. The platform should provide a personalized experience, taking into account each user's unique needs and preferences. By incorporating features such as goal-setting, progress tracking, and reminders, individuals can stay motivated and committed to their health journey.

However, it is important to strike a balance between functionality and simplicity. While it is tempting to include numerous features and options, a cluttered interface can overwhelm users and hinder their ability to navigate and engage effectively. Therefore, designers must prioritize essential features and ensure that the platform remains user-friendly and easy to navigate.

To cater to the diverse needs of internet users, health platforms should also be accessible across various devices, including smartphones, tablets, and computers. This flexibility allows individuals to access their health information and resources whenever and wherever they need them, enhancing the overall convenience and usability of the platform.

In conclusion, the success of internet-based health platforms relies heavily on providing users with an exceptional UI and UX. By creating visually appealing, user-friendly interfaces and incorporating personalized features, these platforms can empower individuals to take control of their health and well-being. As internet users, it is crucial to prioritize our experience and choose platforms that prioritize our needs, ultimately contributing to the digital wellness revolution.

Feedback and Progress Tracking

In today's digital age, the internet has become an integral part of our lives, permeating almost every aspect of our existence. From communication to entertainment and now even health, the internet has revolutionized the way we approach various aspects of our wellbeing. This subchapter explores the significance of feedback and progress tracking in the realm of internet-based health platforms, highlighting their benefits and importance in improving our overall wellness.

Internet-based health platforms have paved the way for a digital wellness revolution, offering individuals the opportunity to take control of their health and well-being from the comfort of their own homes. One key component of these platforms is the ability to receive valuable feedback on our progress. Feedback is crucial as it allows us to understand our strengths and weaknesses, helping us make informed decisions to improve our overall health.

With the help of internet-based health platforms, individuals can track their progress in real-time, giving them a clear picture of their health journey. These platforms provide innovative tools and technologies that enable us to monitor our vital signs, physical activity, sleep patterns, and even mental well-being. By leveraging these tools, we gain valuable insights into our progress, allowing us to make necessary adjustments to our routines and behaviors.

Feedback and progress tracking also play a vital role in motivating individuals to stay on track with their health goals. Whether it's losing weight, improving cardiovascular fitness, or managing stress, the ability to see tangible progress can be a powerful motivator. Internet-based health platforms leverage gamification techniques and personalized feedback to keep users engaged and motivated on their wellness journey.

Furthermore, these platforms enable individuals to connect with a community of like-minded individuals who are on a similar health journey. This sense of community fosters support, encouragement, and accountability, all of which are crucial elements for achieving long-term success.

In conclusion, feedback and progress tracking are essential components of internet-based health platforms. By leveraging these tools, individuals can gain valuable insights into their health journey, make informed decisions, and stay motivated to achieve their wellness goals. Whether you are looking to lose weight, improve fitness, or manage stress, the digital wellness revolution offers a plethora of opportunities to take control of your health and embrace a happier, healthier lifestyle.

Chapter 4: Maximizing Health and Wellness with Digital Platforms

Setting Health Goals

In today's digital age, where the internet plays a significant role in our daily lives, taking charge of our health has become more accessible than ever before. The internet has revolutionized the way we approach healthcare, offering a plethora of online platforms and resources to help us make informed decisions about our well-being. However, with this abundance of information, it can be overwhelming to know where to start. This subchapter aims to guide you through the process of setting health goals using internet-based platforms, regardless of your background or expertise.

Setting health goals is crucial for maintaining overall well-being and achieving a healthier lifestyle. It provides focus, motivation, and a sense of direction. By utilizing internet-based health platforms, you can harness the power of technology to facilitate and track your progress towards these goals.

Firstly, it's essential to identify your specific health goals. Are you looking to lose weight, improve your fitness level, manage stress, or address a chronic condition? Internet-based platforms cater to a wide range of health concerns, offering personalized solutions for each individual.

Once you have identified your goals, the next step is to find the right internet-based health platform that suits your needs. There are numerous platforms available, ranging from fitness apps and nutrition trackers to mental health resources and online support groups. Consider factors such as user-friendliness, credibility, and the features offered by each platform.

After selecting a suitable platform, it's time to create a plan of action. Break your health goals into smaller, achievable targets and determine a timeline for each milestone. Internet-based platforms often provide tools to help you set reminders, track progress, and provide valuable insights into your health journey.

Additionally, take advantage of the online communities and support systems available through these platforms. Engaging with like-minded individuals can provide encouragement, advice, and a sense of accountability. Share your progress, challenges, and successes with others, fostering a supportive network that keeps you motivated.

Remember, setting health goals is not a one-time task but a continuous process. Regularly reassess and adjust your goals as you progress and evolve. The internet-based health platforms of today are dynamic and constantly evolving, allowing you to adapt and refine your goals accordingly.

In conclusion, the internet has revolutionized the way we approach healthcare, making it easier than ever to set and achieve health goals. By utilizing internet-based health platforms, you can customize your approach, track your progress, and connect with others on a similar health journey. Take charge of your well-being and embrace the digital wellness revolution!

Identifying Your Health Priorities

In this digital age, where the internet has become an integral part of our lives, taking charge of our health has never been easier. The internet offers a plethora of health platforms and resources that can revolutionize the way we approach our well-being. However, with so much information and numerous options available, it can be overwhelming to determine where to start. To make the most of the digital wellness revolution, it is crucial to identify your health priorities.

Understanding your health priorities is essential because it allows you to focus your efforts and resources on what matters most. The internet offers a wide range of health-related options, such as fitness apps, online consultations with healthcare professionals, and health tracking devices. By identifying your health priorities, you can narrow down your search and find the tools and platforms that align with your specific needs.

Start by assessing your current health status and determining areas that require attention. Are you looking to lose weight, manage a chronic condition, improve your mental health, or simply maintain overall well-being? Once you have identified your primary health goals, you can search for internet-based health platforms that cater to those specific needs.

Consider your lifestyle and preferences when choosing internet-based health platforms. Do you prefer a structured fitness program that provides workout routines and nutrition plans, or do you enjoy the flexibility of choosing your own activities? Are you more inclined towards guided meditation and stress management apps, or would you benefit from online therapy sessions? The internet offers a wide range of options to suit different preferences, ensuring that you can find a digital wellness solution that is tailored to your individual needs.

Additionally, it is important to consider the credibility and reliability of the platforms you choose. Look for evidence-based information and verified user reviews to ensure that you are making informed decisions about your health. Consult with healthcare professionals or trusted sources to gather recommendations and insights on the most reputable internet-based health platforms available.

Remember that identifying your health priorities is an ongoing process. As your circumstances change and new health goals arise, reassessing your priorities will help you adapt and make the most of the digital wellness revolution. Stay open-minded and explore different internet-based health platforms to find what works best for you. The digital world is full of opportunities to enhance your well-being, and by identifying your health priorities, you can take full advantage of the vast resources available at your fingertips.

Setting Realistic and Measurable Goals

In today's fast-paced digital age, it is easy to get caught up in the endless possibilities and opportunities that the internet offers. With the vast array of health platforms available at our fingertips, it is crucial to set realistic and measurable goals to make the most out of our online experiences and maximize our digital wellness.

Setting goals is an essential aspect of any successful journey, and the world of the internet is no exception. Whether you are seeking to improve your physical fitness, mental well-being, or overall health, setting tangible and achievable goals is the key to staying focused and motivated.

When setting goals in the digital realm, it is crucial to be realistic about what you can accomplish. The internet is a vast space filled with countless resources and options, but it is essential to remember that change takes time. Instead of aiming for drastic transformations overnight, focus on setting small, attainable goals that can be built upon over time. For example, if your goal is to improve your fitness level, start by committing to a certain number of workouts per week and gradually increase the intensity and duration as you progress.

Measurability is another crucial aspect of setting goals in the digital world. With the abundance of health platforms available, it is easier than ever to track your progress and measure your achievements. Utilize the various tracking tools and apps to monitor your physical activity, sleep patterns, or even your nutrition intake. By having concrete data on your progress, you can better assess your strengths and areas for improvement, making it easier to set new goals and track your success.

It is important to remember that everyone's journey is unique, and what works for one person may not work for another. Therefore, it is essential to set goals that are tailored to your individual needs and capabilities. Take into account your current lifestyle, commitments, and limitations when setting your goals, ensuring that they are realistic and achievable within your circumstances.

In conclusion, setting realistic and measurable goals is a fundamental step in maximizing your digital wellness. By setting achievable targets and utilizing the vast resources available on the internet, you can harness the power of technology to enhance your overall health and well-being. Remember to be patient, track your progress, and customize your goals to suit your individual needs. Embrace the digital wellness revolution and unlock your full potential in the internet age.

Leveraging Digital Tools for Exercise and Nutrition

In today's digital age, the internet has transformed almost every aspect of our lives, including how we approach health and wellness. With an abundance of information and resources available at our fingertips, it has become easier than ever to leverage digital tools for exercise and nutrition. Whether you are a fitness enthusiast, someone looking to improve their overall well-being, or even a beginner just starting on their wellness journey, the internet offers a wealth of platforms and applications to support your goals.

One of the key advantages of utilizing digital tools for exercise and nutrition is the accessibility they provide. No longer do you need to rely solely on expensive gym memberships or personal trainers. With a simple internet connection, you can access a wide range of workout routines, exercise videos, and fitness apps that cater to all fitness levels and goals. From high-intensity interval training (HIIT) programs to yoga sessions and everything in between, there is something for everyone.

Moreover, digital tools can also offer personalized nutrition guidance. Gone are the days of sifting through countless diet books or consulting with nutritionists. Online platforms and mobile apps now allow you to track your food intake, count calories, and even provide recommendations based on your specific dietary needs and goals. This level of personalization and convenience enables you to make informed choices about your nutrition and stay accountable to your health goals.

Additionally, the internet provides a supportive community for individuals interested in exercise and nutrition. Social media platforms, online forums, and fitness communities allow you to connect with like-minded individuals, share your progress, and seek advice from experts. These virtual communities can provide motivation, inspiration, and a sense of belonging, creating a supportive environment that helps you stay committed to your health and wellness journey.

However, it is important to approach digital tools for exercise and nutrition with caution. With the vast amount of information available online, it is crucial to ensure that the sources you rely on are credible and evidence-based. Always consult with healthcare professionals or certified trainers before making any significant changes to your exercise or nutrition routine.

In conclusion, the digital revolution has opened up endless possibilities for leveraging digital tools to support exercise and nutrition. Whether you are a fitness enthusiast or someone just starting on their wellness journey, the internet offers a wealth of resources to help you achieve your health goals. From workout routines and fitness apps to personalized nutrition guidance and virtual communities, the digital landscape has transformed the way we approach our well-being, making it more accessible, personalized, and supportive than ever before. So, embrace the digital tools available to you and embark on a journey towards a healthier, happier you.

Finding the Right Fitness App or Program

In today's digital age, the internet has revolutionized every aspect of our lives, including our health and wellness. With the rise of fitness apps and programs, it has become easier than ever to stay active and make positive changes to our physical well-being. However, with so many options available, it can be overwhelming to find the right fitness app or program that suits our individual needs and goals. This subchapter aims to guide you through the process of finding the perfect fitness app or program for you in the vast realm of the internet.

First and foremost, it is essential to identify your fitness goals. Are you looking to lose weight, build muscle, improve flexibility, or simply lead a healthier lifestyle? Understanding your objectives will help narrow down the options and focus on apps or programs that cater specifically to your needs. Different fitness apps offer various features, such as personalized workout plans, nutrition tracking, or mindfulness exercises. Identifying which features align with your goals will help you make an informed decision.

Next, consider your level of expertise and fitness experience. Some apps or programs are designed for beginners, while others target more advanced users. It is crucial to find an app or program that matches your fitness level to ensure both safety and effectiveness. Many fitness apps provide detailed descriptions and user reviews, which can give you valuable insights into the app's suitability for your specific fitness level.

Another important factor to consider is the app's user interface and overall user experience. A well-designed app with an intuitive interface can greatly enhance your fitness journey. Look for apps that are easy to navigate, visually appealing, and offer a seamless user experience. Reading user testimonials and reviews can give you a sense of whether an app is user-friendly and enjoyable to use.

Lastly, consider the cost and commitment required by the app or program. Some fitness apps offer free versions with limited features, while others require a subscription or one-time payment for full access. It is crucial to evaluate your budget and determine how much you are willing to invest in a fitness app or program. Additionally, consider the time commitment required by the app or program. Some apps may require a significant time commitment, while others offer shorter, more flexible workouts.

In conclusion, finding the right fitness app or program in the wide array of options available on the internet can be a daunting task. By identifying your fitness goals, considering your fitness level, evaluating the user interface, and assessing the cost and commitment required, you can make an informed decision that will maximize your fitness journey. Remember, the right fitness app or program is the one that aligns with your specific needs, motivates you, and keeps you engaged on your path to a healthier lifestyle.

Tracking and Analyzing Nutritional Intake

In today's digital age, where the internet has become an integral part of our lives, it is no surprise that it has also revolutionized the way we approach health and wellness. With the advent of internet-based health platforms, individuals now have access to a plethora of tools and resources to monitor and improve their overall well-being. One such tool is the ability to track and analyze nutritional intake, which plays a vital role in maintaining a healthy lifestyle.

Internet-based health platforms offer a wide range of applications and websites that allow users to easily track their nutritional intake. These platforms provide a comprehensive database of food items, including their nutritional content, making it easier than ever to keep track of what we consume. Whether you are looking to lose weight, manage a specific health condition, or simply improve your overall health, tracking your nutritional intake can be a game-changer.

By monitoring your nutritional intake through these platforms, you gain a deeper understanding of the nutrients you are consuming and can make more informed choices about your diet. From macronutrients like carbohydrates, proteins, and fats to micronutrients like vitamins and minerals, these platforms provide detailed insights into the nutritional value of the foods you consume. This information allows you to identify areas of improvement and make necessary adjustments to optimize your diet.

Moreover, tracking your nutritional intake can also help you identify patterns and trends in your eating habits. Are you consuming too much sugar? Are you getting enough fiber? These platforms often offer visual representations of your data, such as graphs and charts, which make it easier to identify areas of concern. Armed with this knowledge, you can make conscious decisions to modify your diet and improve your overall health.

Furthermore, internet-based health platforms often offer additional features such as meal planning and recipe suggestions based on your nutritional goals. These tools can help you create balanced meal plans that meet your specific dietary needs and preferences. Whether you are following a specific diet plan or have unique nutritional requirements, these platforms can assist you in achieving your health goals.

In conclusion, tracking and analyzing nutritional intake has been made convenient and accessible through internet-based health platforms. By utilizing these tools, individuals can gain valuable insights into their dietary habits and make informed decisions to improve their overall well-being. Whether you are looking to lose weight, manage a health condition, or simply lead a healthier lifestyle, tracking your nutritional intake is a key step in optimizing your health. Embrace the digital wellness revolution and take control of your nutrition today!

Utilizing Telemedicine for Remote Care

In today's digital age, the internet has revolutionized various aspects of our lives, including healthcare. The emergence of telemedicine has provided an innovative solution to bridge the gap between patients and healthcare professionals, especially for those who are unable to access traditional healthcare services. This subchapter explores the incredible potential of telemedicine and how it has transformed remote care.

Telemedicine refers to the use of technology, particularly the internet, to deliver healthcare services remotely. Through telemedicine, patients can connect with healthcare providers through video consultations, online messaging, or phone calls. This convenience eliminates the need for in-person visits, making healthcare accessible to individuals residing in remote areas or facing mobility challenges.

One of the primary advantages of telemedicine is its ability to provide immediate care, regardless of physical distance. With just a stable internet connection, patients can receive medical advice, prescriptions, and follow-up care from the comfort of their own homes. This not only saves time and money but also ensures that patients receive prompt attention, leading to better health outcomes.

Telemedicine has proven particularly beneficial in rural communities, where access to specialized medical services can be limited. Specialists can now reach patients virtually, reducing the need for long and expensive journeys. Moreover, telemedicine has played a crucial role in emergency situations, enabling healthcare professionals to provide remote guidance and assistance until the patient can receive in-person care.

Furthermore, telemedicine has significantly improved healthcare access for individuals with chronic conditions. By monitoring vital signs and symptoms through wearable devices, healthcare providers can remotely track patients' progress and intervene when necessary. This proactive approach promotes self-management and empowers patients to take control of their health, reducing hospital readmissions and overall healthcare costs.

The internet's role in telemedicine extends beyond patient-doctor interactions. It has facilitated the exchange of electronic health records, allowing healthcare professionals to access and share patient information seamlessly. This interoperability enhances care coordination and ensures that patients receive comprehensive and personalized treatment, regardless of geographical barriers.

In conclusion, telemedicine has emerged as a game-changer in remote care, revolutionizing the way healthcare is delivered. The internet has paved the way for convenient, immediate, and accessible healthcare services, benefiting individuals across various demographics, including those in rural areas. With the continued advancements in technology, telemedicine holds immense potential to further improve health outcomes and transform the delivery of healthcare worldwide.

Accessing Virtual Doctor Consultations

In today's digital age, the internet has revolutionized almost every aspect of our lives, and the field of healthcare is no exception. With the increasing popularity of internet-based health platforms, accessing virtual doctor consultations has become a convenient and efficient way to receive medical advice and treatment. This subchapter will explore the benefits and considerations of accessing virtual doctor consultations, shedding light on how this innovative approach to healthcare can empower individuals in taking control of their well-being.

One of the key advantages of virtual doctor consultations is the convenience it offers. Gone are the days of waiting for hours in a crowded waiting room, only to spend a few minutes face-to-face with a doctor. With the click of a button, individuals can now connect with healthcare professionals from the comfort of their own homes. This not only saves valuable time but also eliminates the need for travel, making it especially beneficial for those living in remote areas or with limited mobility.

Furthermore, virtual doctor consultations provide a level of accessibility that was previously unimaginable. Through internet-based health platforms, individuals can easily access healthcare services regardless of their location, socioeconomic status, or physical abilities. This inclusivity ensures that everyone has the opportunity to receive the medical attention they need, promoting equity and equal opportunities for better health.

However, it is important to consider the limitations and potential challenges of accessing virtual doctor consultations. While this method is suitable for many non-emergency medical concerns, it may not be appropriate for all situations. Some conditions require in-person examinations, diagnostic tests, or emergency interventions that cannot be adequately addressed through virtual consultations alone. Therefore, it is crucial to understand the scope and limitations of virtual consultations and use them as a complement to traditional healthcare, rather than a replacement.

In conclusion, accessing virtual doctor consultations through internet-based health platforms has revolutionized the way we approach healthcare. The convenience, accessibility, and inclusivity offered by this innovative approach empower individuals to take control of their well-being and seek medical advice and treatment with ease. However, it is important to understand the limitations and use virtual consultations as a complementary tool alongside traditional healthcare practices. By embracing the digital wellness revolution, we can maximize the benefits of internet-based health platforms and improve the overall health and wellness of individuals worldwide.

Remote Monitoring and Chronic Disease Management

In today's digital era, the internet has revolutionized various aspects of our lives, and healthcare is no exception. The advent of internet-based health platforms has opened up new possibilities for managing chronic diseases remotely. This subchapter explores the transformative potential of remote monitoring in chronic disease management and its impact on improving the overall well-being of individuals.

Chronic diseases such as diabetes, hypertension, and asthma affect millions of people worldwide. Traditionally, managing these conditions required frequent visits to healthcare providers, leading to inconvenience and increased healthcare costs. However, with the rise of internet-based health platforms, individuals can now monitor their chronic diseases from the comfort of their homes using various digital tools.

Remote monitoring enables individuals to track their vital signs, medication adherence, and disease progression in real-time. Wearable devices, such as smartwatches and fitness trackers, can collect data on heart rate, blood pressure, and blood glucose levels, providing valuable insights for individuals and healthcare professionals alike. This continuous monitoring allows for early detection of any deviations from normal values, enabling timely interventions and preventing complications.

Internet-based health platforms also facilitate seamless communication between patients and healthcare providers. Through secure messaging systems or video consultations, individuals can consult with their healthcare team, discuss their concerns, and receive guidance on managing their chronic conditions effectively. This enhances patient engagement, improves treatment adherence, and empowers individuals to take charge of their health.

Moreover, remote monitoring enables personalized care plans based on individual needs. By analyzing the collected data, healthcare professionals can gain a comprehensive understanding of each patient's condition, enabling tailored interventions and adjustments to treatment plans. This individualized approach improves outcomes and reduces hospitalizations.

For the internet niche, these digital health platforms offer a wealth of information and resources at the click of a button. Internet users can access educational materials, self-management tools, and support communities specific to their chronic conditions. This empowers individuals to become proactive participants in their healthcare journey, leading to better health outcomes and improved quality of life.

In conclusion, remote monitoring through internet-based health platforms has revolutionized chronic disease management. It empowers individuals to monitor their conditions, facilitates efficient communication with healthcare providers, and promotes personalized care plans. For internet users, these platforms provide an abundance of knowledge and support. The digital wellness revolution has transformed the way we manage chronic diseases, offering a brighter and healthier future for everyone.

Promoting Mental Health and Well-being Online

In today's digital age, the internet has become an integral part of our lives. It has revolutionized the way we communicate, work, and access information. With the advent of internet-based health platforms, individuals now have the opportunity to promote their mental health and well-being online like never before. This subchapter aims to explore the various ways in which the internet can be utilized to enhance mental health and well-being, catering to individuals from all walks of life.

The internet offers a plethora of resources and tools that can be harnessed to promote mental health and well-being. From online therapy platforms to mental health apps, people can now access professional help and guidance from the comfort of their own homes. Online therapy platforms provide a convenient and affordable alternative to traditional face-to-face therapy sessions. They enable individuals to connect with licensed therapists through secure video calls, chat, or email, ensuring privacy and confidentiality.

Additionally, the internet serves as a valuable source of information and support for those seeking to improve their mental health. Online communities and forums dedicated to mental health provide a safe space for individuals to share their experiences, seek advice, and connect with others who may be going through similar challenges. These platforms foster a sense of belonging and support, reducing feelings of isolation and promoting overall well-being.

Furthermore, internet-based health platforms can offer a wide range of self-help resources, such as guided meditation apps, stress management techniques, and mindfulness exercises. These tools empower individuals to take control of their mental health and develop coping strategies to navigate life's challenges effectively.

However, it is essential to approach internet-based mental health resources with caution. The vastness of the internet means that not all information and resources available online are accurate or reliable. It is crucial for individuals to rely on reputable sources and consult professionals when necessary. Additionally, maintaining a healthy balance between online and offline activities is crucial to prevent excessive screen time and potential negative effects on mental health.

In conclusion, the internet has opened up a world of possibilities for promoting mental health and well-being. From accessing professional help online to connecting with supportive communities and utilizing self-help resources, the internet offers a wealth of tools and information to enhance mental well-being. However, it is important to use these resources responsibly, ensuring that individuals seek reputable sources and maintain a healthy balance between online and offline activities. By harnessing the power of the internet, individuals can take proactive steps towards improving their mental health and overall well-being.

Exploring Meditation and Mindfulness Apps

In today's fast-paced digital world, finding moments of peace and tranquility can be a challenge. However, thanks to the rise of meditation and mindfulness apps, harnessing the power of technology for personal well-being has become more accessible than ever before. These apps offer a range of tools and techniques to help individuals cultivate mindfulness, reduce stress, and achieve a state of inner calm.

Meditation apps have gained immense popularity due to their convenience and effectiveness in promoting mental and emotional well-being. With just a few taps on your smartphone, you can access a vast library of guided meditations, breathing exercises, and calming music. Whether you are a beginner or an experienced meditator, these apps provide a wealth of resources to support your practice.

Mindfulness apps, on the other hand, focus on bringing awareness to the present moment and fostering a non-judgmental attitude towards one's thoughts and emotions. These apps often offer features like daily reminders, gratitude journals, and mindful exercises to help users stay grounded and connected to themselves and their surroundings.

The internet has played a significant role in the growth of these meditation and mindfulness apps. With the power of the internet, these platforms have been able to reach a global audience, allowing individuals from all walks of life to embark on their wellness journey. Whether you live in a bustling city or a remote village, all you need is an internet connection to access these transformative tools.

Moreover, the internet has facilitated the creation of online communities and forums dedicated to meditation and mindfulness, where users can connect, share their experiences, and seek guidance from experts. These virtual spaces provide a sense of belonging and support, reminding us that we are not alone in our pursuit of well-being.

However, as with any digital platform, it is essential to approach meditation and mindfulness apps mindfully. While these apps can be powerful tools for self-discovery and personal growth, it is crucial to strike a balance between digital engagement and real-world experiences. It is advisable to use these apps as a complement to your offline practice and seek guidance from qualified professionals when needed.

In conclusion, meditation and mindfulness apps offer a gateway to a world of serenity and self-discovery in the digital age. With the internet as our ally, we can reap the benefits of these transformative practices, no matter where we are. By exploring these apps, we can cultivate a sense of inner calm and enhance our overall well-being in the midst of our internet-dominated lives.

Connecting with Online Support Communities

Subchapter: Connecting with Online Support Communities

In this digital age, the internet has become an integral part of our lives. It has opened up numerous possibilities and has revolutionized the way we connect and communicate with others. One of the most significant aspects of the internet is the emergence of online support communities. These virtual spaces have transformed the way we seek and receive support, guidance, and information.

Online support communities provide a unique platform for individuals to connect with others who share similar experiences, challenges, or interests. Whether you are facing a health issue, struggling with mental health, seeking advice on parenting, or looking for support in any other aspect of your life, there is likely an online community waiting to welcome you.

The internet has made it easier than ever to find and join these communities. With just a few clicks, you can connect with people from all over the world who can relate to your situation. These communities offer a safe and non-judgmental space where you can share your thoughts, concerns, and experiences, knowing that others will understand and empathize.

Not only do online support communities provide emotional support, but they also offer a wealth of knowledge and resources. Members often share information, tips, and strategies that they have found helpful in dealing with their own challenges. This collective wisdom can be invaluable in navigating various aspects of life, be it managing a chronic illness, learning new skills, or finding ways to improve your overall well-being.

Moreover, online support communities foster a sense of belonging and empowerment. They can help you realize that you are not alone in your struggles and that there are others who have overcome similar obstacles. By connecting with like-minded individuals, you can gain inspiration, motivation, and a renewed sense of hope.

However, it is important to approach online support communities with caution. While most communities are genuine and supportive, it is essential to verify the credibility and reliability of the information shared. Always consult a healthcare professional or trusted source when seeking medical advice or making important decisions about your health.

In conclusion, online support communities have transformed the way we connect, seek support, and share knowledge. The internet has made it possible for individuals from all walks of life to come together, support one another, and build meaningful relationships. Whether you are looking for emotional support, practical advice, or simply a place to belong, online support communities offer a world of opportunities for everyone navigating the vast landscape of the internet. Embrace this digital revolution and discover the power of connecting with others in online support communities.

Chapter 5: Overcoming Challenges and Ensuring Digital Wellbeing

Privacy and Security Concerns

In today's digital era, where the internet plays a significant role in our lives, it is crucial to address the privacy and security concerns that accompany this growing dependence on internet-based health platforms. While the internet has revolutionized the way we access and manage our health information, it also brings forth potential risks that need to be acknowledged and addressed.

One of the primary concerns regarding privacy on internet-based health platforms is the vulnerability of personal data. When we share our health-related information online, we expose ourselves to the possibility of unauthorized access or data breaches. This could lead to severe consequences, such as identity theft, financial fraud, or misuse of sensitive health records. Therefore, it is essential to choose platforms that prioritize data protection and employ robust security measures to safeguard personal information.

Moreover, privacy concerns arise from the collection and use of personal data by internet-based health platforms. Many platforms gather user data to improve their services, target advertisements, or even sell the data to third parties. This raises ethical questions regarding the ownership and control of personal health information. Users must have control over their data and be aware of how it is being used to make informed decisions about their privacy.

To address these concerns, it is crucial for internet-based health platforms to adopt strict privacy policies and transparent data practices. Users should be provided with clear information about data collection, storage, and sharing practices. Additionally, platforms should offer robust security measures, such as encryption and secure data storage, to protect user information from unauthorized access.

As individuals, it is also our responsibility to take steps to protect our privacy and security online. This includes using strong and unique passwords, being mindful of the information we share, and being cautious about the platforms we choose to engage with. Regularly reviewing privacy settings and keeping software and antivirus programs up to date can also contribute to maintaining a secure online presence.

Overall, while internet-based health platforms offer numerous benefits, it is essential for users and platform providers to prioritize privacy and security. By being aware of the potential risks and taking appropriate measures, we can maximize the benefits of these platforms while safeguarding our personal information. The digital wellness revolution can only flourish if privacy and security concerns are adequately addressed, ensuring a trusted and safe environment for everyone on the internet.

Protecting Personal Health Information

In the era of digital wellness, where internet-based health platforms have become an integral part of our lives, it is crucial to understand the significance of protecting personal health information. With the vast amount of sensitive data being shared and stored online, it is essential for everyone, regardless of their background or expertise, to be aware of the potential risks and take necessary measures to safeguard their personal health information.

The internet has undoubtedly revolutionized the healthcare industry, offering numerous benefits such as easy access to medical records, telemedicine consultations, and personalized health recommendations. However, this convenience comes with the responsibility of protecting our personal health information from unauthorized access and potential breaches.

One of the primary steps in safeguarding personal health information is to choose reputable and secure internet-based health platforms. When selecting a platform, it is crucial to consider factors such as privacy policies, encryption measures, and data storage practices. Opting for platforms that comply with industry standards and regulations, like Health Insurance Portability and Accountability Act (HIPAA) in the United States, ensures that your personal health information is handled securely.

Additionally, users should proactively manage their privacy settings on internet-based health platforms. Many platforms offer customizable privacy settings that allow individuals to control the accessibility of their personal health information. By carefully reviewing and adjusting these settings, users can limit the exposure of their data and ensure that only authorized individuals or healthcare professionals have access to it.

Regularly updating passwords and enabling two-factor authentication is another vital aspect of protecting personal health information. Strong and unique passwords, along with additional layers of authentication, add an extra level of security to prevent unauthorized access to health-related data.

Furthermore, individuals should remain vigilant against phishing attempts, malware, and other cyber threats. Educating oneself about common online scams and practicing safe browsing habits, such as avoiding suspicious links and downloading from trusted sources, can significantly reduce the risk of falling victim to cyberattacks.

In conclusion, protecting personal health information is paramount in the digital wellness revolution. By choosing secure platforms, managing privacy settings, updating passwords, and staying informed about online threats, individuals can ensure the confidentiality and integrity of their personal health information. Through these proactive measures, we can fully embrace the benefits of internet-based health platforms while minimizing potential risks in an increasingly interconnected world.

Evaluating Platform Security Measures

In today's digital age, the internet has revolutionized the way we access and manage our health. With the emergence of internet-based health platforms, individuals now have the ability to monitor their well-being, connect with healthcare professionals, and access a vast array of health-related information anytime, anywhere. However, with these benefits come concerns about the security and privacy of our personal health data. This subchapter aims to provide valuable insights on how to evaluate platform security measures to ensure a safe and secure online healthcare experience.

When it comes to evaluating platform security measures, there are several key factors to consider. Firstly, it is crucial to assess the platform's data encryption protocols. Encryption is a process that converts sensitive information into unreadable code, making it virtually impossible for unauthorized individuals to access or decipher. Look for platforms that utilize strong encryption algorithms, such as Advanced Encryption Standard (AES) 256-bit, which is widely recognized as highly secure.

Another important aspect to consider is the platform's authentication and access controls. Robust authentication measures, such as two-factor authentication, provide an additional layer of security by requiring users to provide two forms of identification (e.g., password and a unique code sent to their mobile device) before granting access to their accounts. Additionally, the platform should employ strict access controls, ensuring that only authorized individuals have access to sensitive health data.

Furthermore, it is essential to evaluate the platform's data storage and backup practices. Look for platforms that store data in highly secure data centers equipped with advanced physical and virtual security measures, such as firewalls, intrusion detection systems, and round-the-clock surveillance. Regular data backups should also be conducted to prevent data loss in case of unforeseen events or system failures.

Additionally, consider the platform's compliance with industry standards and regulations. Healthcare platforms should adhere to strict regulations, such as the Health Insurance Portability and Accountability Act (HIPAA) in the United States. Compliance with such regulations ensures that your personal health data is handled and protected in accordance with the highest security standards.

Lastly, don't forget to review the platform's privacy policy and terms of service. Look for platforms that clearly outline how they collect, store, and use your data. Transparency is key when it comes to online platforms, and understanding how your data is being handled will help you make informed decisions about your digital wellness journey.

In conclusion, evaluating platform security measures is crucial for ensuring a safe and secure online healthcare experience. By considering factors such as data encryption, authentication and access controls, data storage practices, compliance with regulations, and transparency in privacy policies, individuals can make informed decisions when choosing an internet-based health platform. Prioritizing platform security will enable everyone to maximize the benefits of the digital wellness revolution while safeguarding their personal health information.

Addressing Digital Addiction

In today's hyper-connected world, the internet has become an integral part of our lives. It has revolutionized the way we communicate, work, and access information. However, with the increasing reliance on digital devices and online platforms, a new challenge has emerged – digital addiction. This subchapter explores the concept of digital addiction and provides practical strategies to address this growing issue.

Digital addiction refers to the excessive and compulsive use of digital devices, such as smartphones, tablets, and computers. It affects individuals from all walks of life and can have severe consequences on physical and mental well-being. Internet addiction can lead to social isolation, sleep disturbances, decreased productivity, and even mental health disorders like depression and anxiety.

To address digital addiction, it is important to develop a healthy relationship with technology. Here are some strategies that can help:

1. Awareness and self-reflection: Recognize and acknowledge your digital habits. Take a moment to reflect on how much time you spend online and whether it is interfering with other aspects of your life.

2. Set boundaries: Establish clear boundaries for screen time. Allocate specific periods for using digital devices and make sure to disconnect during important activities such as meals, family time, or before bedtime.

3. Digital detox: Take regular breaks from the digital world. Engage in offline activities, hobbies, and spend quality time with loved ones to recharge and rejuvenate.

4. Practice mindful internet use: Be conscious of your online activities. Avoid mindless scrolling and focus on purposeful engagement. Prioritize productive and meaningful online interactions.

5. Seek support: If you find it challenging to control your digital usage, seek support from friends, family, or professionals. There are numerous resources available, such as support groups, therapy, or digital wellness apps.

6. Create a tech-friendly environment: Make your living space or workplace conducive to digital wellness. Set up designated tech-free zones and limit distractions to enhance focus and reduce the temptation to indulge in excessive screen time.

Addressing digital addiction is crucial for maintaining a healthy and balanced life in the digital age. By adopting these strategies, you can regain control over your digital habits and maximize the benefits of the internet while minimizing its negative impact on your well-being.

Remember, the internet is a powerful tool that can enhance our lives, but it is essential to maintain a healthy balance to ensure optimal digital wellness.

Recognizing the Signs of Digital Addiction

In today's digital age, the internet has become an integral part of our daily lives. From social media platforms to online shopping and information seeking, the internet offers endless possibilities and conveniences. However, with the increasing reliance on the digital world, it's essential to be aware of the signs of digital addiction, as it can have serious consequences on our mental and physical well-being.

Digital addiction, also known as internet addiction, refers to the compulsive and excessive use of digital devices and online activities. It can manifest in various forms, including excessive use of social media, gaming, video streaming, online gambling, and even constant checking of emails and notifications. While it may seem harmless at first, digital addiction can gradually take over our lives, leading to negative impacts on our relationships, work, and overall health.

One of the key signs to watch out for is an overwhelming preoccupation with digital activities. If you find yourself constantly thinking about the next time you can go online or feeling anxious when you're unable to access the internet, it may be a red flag. Another indicator is neglecting important responsibilities or activities in favor of spending more time online. If you find that your online activities are causing you to miss deadlines, neglect personal relationships, or neglect self-care, it may be time to reassess your digital habits.

Physical symptoms can also be warning signs of digital addiction. Spending excessive time in front of screens can lead to eye strain, headaches, and disrupted sleep patterns. If you notice these symptoms worsening or becoming persistent, it's crucial to address the underlying issue. Additionally, changes in mood, such as irritability, restlessness, or depression when unable to engage in digital activities, can indicate a problem.

Recognizing the signs of digital addiction is the first step towards regaining control over our relationship with the internet. It is essential to set boundaries and establish healthy habits when it comes to our digital consumption. This could include limiting screen time, scheduling regular breaks, and engaging in offline activities that bring joy and fulfillment.

Remember, the internet is a powerful tool that can enhance our lives, but it should not consume us. By recognizing the signs of digital addiction and taking proactive steps to maintain a healthy balance, we can fully embrace the benefits of the digital world while safeguarding our well-being.

Implementing Healthy Digital Habits

In today's interconnected world, the internet plays a central role in our lives. It has revolutionized the way we communicate, work, and access information. However, with the widespread use of internet-based platforms, it is crucial to develop healthy digital habits to ensure our overall well-being. This subchapter explores effective strategies to implement healthy digital habits and maximize the benefits of the internet while minimizing its potential drawbacks.

1. Mindful Internet Usage: The first step in implementing healthy digital habits is to be mindful of our internet usage. Often, we find ourselves mindlessly scrolling through social media or spending countless hours online without realizing it. By being aware of our online activities, we can consciously allocate time for productive tasks and limit unnecessary internet browsing.

2. Set Boundaries: Establishing clear boundaries around internet usage is essential. Determine specific time limits for various online activities, such as work-related tasks, social media, and entertainment. Setting boundaries allows us to maintain a healthy balance between our digital and offline lives, ensuring that the internet does not consume all our time and attention.

3. Practice Digital Detox: Regularly disconnecting from the online world through a digital detox is crucial for our mental well-being. Designate specific periods, such as weekends or evenings, to disconnect entirely from the internet. Engage in activities that promote relaxation and rejuvenation, such as reading a book, spending time in nature, or pursuing a hobby.

4. Prioritize Real-life Connections: While the internet offers numerous opportunities for virtual connections, it is essential to prioritize real-life relationships. Engage in face-to-face interactions, plan outings with friends and family, and participate in community activities. Building strong offline connections provides a sense of belonging and fulfillment that cannot be replicated online.

5. Protect Digital Privacy: Safeguarding our digital privacy is crucial in maintaining healthy digital habits. Be cautious about sharing personal information online and regularly review privacy settings on social media platforms. Utilize strong passwords and enable two-factor authentication to protect sensitive data from potential cyber threats.

6. Foster Digital Well-being: Actively seek out internet-based platforms that promote physical and mental well-being. Explore health-related apps, fitness trackers, and online communities that encourage healthy lifestyle choices. Engage in online mindfulness or meditation programs to reduce stress and enhance overall well-being.

By implementing these healthy digital habits, we can reap the benefits of the internet while minimizing its potential negative impacts. Remember, the internet should be a tool that enhances our lives rather than dominating them. Let us embrace the digital wellness revolution and harness the power of the internet to lead happier, healthier, and more fulfilling lives.

Bridging the Digital Divide

In today's digital age, the internet has become an integral part of our lives. It has revolutionized the way we communicate, access information, and even manage our health. However, there is a significant portion of the population that is left behind in this technological boom. This gap between those who have access to the internet and those who don't is known as the digital divide.

The digital divide is a complex issue that affects various aspects of society, including healthcare. As internet-based health platforms become increasingly popular, it is crucial to address this divide to ensure that everyone can benefit from the digital wellness revolution.

One of the main barriers to bridging the digital divide is the lack of internet access in certain communities. Many low-income areas and rural regions still struggle with limited or no internet connectivity. This lack of access not only hinders individuals from accessing vital health information but also prevents them from taking advantage of online health platforms and telemedicine services.

To address this issue, governments and organizations must work together to improve internet infrastructure in underserved areas. Initiatives like providing subsidies for internet service providers, establishing community centers with free internet access, and investing in broadband expansion projects can go a long way in narrowing the digital divide.

Another aspect of the digital divide is the lack of digital literacy among certain demographics. While internet access may be available, some individuals may not possess the necessary skills to navigate online platforms effectively. This digital illiteracy can prevent them from utilizing internet-based health resources and services.

To tackle this problem, educational programs should be implemented to teach people how to use the internet and leverage digital health platforms. These programs can be conducted in schools, community centers, or even through online tutorials. By empowering individuals with digital literacy skills, we can ensure that everyone can participate in the digital wellness revolution.

Moreover, addressing the digital divide also requires making internet-based health platforms more accessible and user-friendly. Developers should place emphasis on creating user interfaces that are intuitive, inclusive, and cater to individuals with varying levels of digital proficiency. Additionally, providing multilingual options and ensuring compatibility with different devices can further enhance accessibility.

Bridging the digital divide is not just an ethical imperative; it is also a necessity for creating a healthier and more equitable society. By ensuring that everyone has access to internet-based health platforms, we can empower individuals to take control of their well-being, improve health outcomes, and reduce healthcare disparities.

In conclusion, the digital divide poses significant challenges in the realm of internet-based health platforms. However, through efforts to improve internet access, digital literacy, and platform accessibility, we can bridge this divide and bring the benefits of the digital wellness revolution to every individual, regardless of their internet niche.

Accessibility and Inclusivity in Internet-based Health Platforms

In the era of technology and the Internet, health platforms have emerged as powerful tools to enhance our overall well-being. Internet-based health platforms offer a wide range of services, such as telemedicine, online consultations, and health monitoring apps, that have revolutionized the way we approach our healthcare needs. However, it is important to recognize that these platforms should be accessible and inclusive for everyone, regardless of their abilities or limitations.

Accessibility in internet-based health platforms refers to designing and developing platforms in a way that enables individuals with disabilities to fully participate and benefit from their services. This includes ensuring that the platforms are compatible with assistive technologies, such as screen readers or voice recognition software, which enable individuals with visual or physical impairments to navigate and interact with the platforms effectively.

Moreover, internet-based health platforms should also prioritize inclusivity. Inclusivity means addressing the diverse needs and preferences of individuals, particularly those from marginalized communities. This includes providing multilingual options, culturally sensitive content, and considerations for individuals with low health literacy or limited access to technology.

Ensuring accessibility and inclusivity in internet-based health platforms not only benefits individuals with disabilities or specific needs, but it also promotes a more equitable and patient-centered healthcare system overall. By embracing accessibility and inclusivity, these platforms can reach a broader audience and enhance the health outcomes for everyone.

To achieve accessibility and inclusivity, developers and designers should adopt universal design principles. Universal design involves creating products and services that are usable by the widest possible range of individuals, regardless of their age, abilities, or disabilities. By incorporating features like adjustable font sizes, clear and simple user interfaces, and providing alternative formats for content, internet-based health platforms can accommodate the needs of a diverse user base.

In conclusion, accessibility and inclusivity are crucial aspects of internet-based health platforms. By ensuring that these platforms are accessible to individuals with disabilities and inclusive of diverse user needs, we can maximize their potential to improve overall wellness for everyone. Through the adoption of universal design principles, we can create a digital wellness revolution that truly benefits every individual, regardless of their internet usage or niche.

In today's digital age, the internet has become an essential part of our lives, revolutionizing the way we access information and interact with others. The internet has also played a significant role in the healthcare industry, providing people with convenient and accessible platforms to manage their health and well-being. However, it is crucial to ensure that these internet-based health platforms are accessible and inclusive to all individuals, regardless of their abilities or backgrounds.

Accessibility is the key to ensuring that everyone can benefit from these platforms. Internet-based health platforms should be designed in a way that accommodates individuals with disabilities, such as visual impairments, hearing impairments, or mobility limitations. This can be achieved by implementing features like screen readers, closed captioning, and keyboard navigation options. By making these platforms accessible, individuals with disabilities can easily navigate and utilize the resources available to improve their health and well-being.

Inclusivity goes beyond accessibility and focuses on providing equal opportunities for individuals from diverse backgrounds. Internet-based health platforms should be culturally sensitive and considerate of the unique needs and preferences of different communities. This involves offering content in multiple languages, incorporating diverse perspectives, and addressing the specific health concerns of various ethnic groups. By embracing inclusivity, these platforms can bridge the gap in healthcare disparities and ensure that everyone has equal access to vital health information and resources.

Moreover, these internet-based health platforms need to address the digital divide, which refers to the gap between individuals who have access to the internet and those who do not. While the internet has become increasingly accessible, there are still many individuals, especially in underserved communities, who lack access to reliable internet connections or digital devices. To overcome this barrier, initiatives should be implemented to provide internet access and digital literacy training to those who are unable to afford or access these resources. By doing so, we can ensure that internet-based health platforms reach as many people as possible and promote health equity.

In conclusion, accessibility and inclusivity are crucial aspects of internet-based health platforms. By designing these platforms with accessibility in mind, considering the unique needs of individuals with disabilities, and embracing inclusivity by catering to diverse communities, we can maximize the potential of these platforms to improve the health and well-being of everyone. It is essential to address the digital divide to ensure that these platforms are accessible to all, regardless of their socioeconomic background. By prioritizing accessibility and inclusivity, we can truly revolutionize the way we approach digital wellness and create a healthier, more equitable world for all.

As the digital revolution continues to transform various aspects of our lives, the internet has become an essential tool for individuals seeking health information, resources, and support. Internet-based health platforms have emerged as a convenient and accessible way to connect with healthcare providers, access medical records, and engage in self-care. However, it is crucial to ensure that these platforms are designed with accessibility and inclusivity in mind to cater to the diverse needs of all users.

In today's interconnected world, the internet has become a lifeline for many individuals who face physical limitations or disabilities. Internet-based health platforms have the potential to empower these individuals by providing them with the means to access vital health information and services. It is essential for developers and designers to prioritize accessibility features such as screen reader compatibility, alternative text for images, and keyboard navigation. By doing so, they can ensure that everyone, regardless of their abilities, can have equal access to these platforms.

Moreover, inclusivity in internet-based health platforms should extend beyond physical disabilities. It is crucial to consider the diverse range of users who may have different cultural backgrounds, languages, or literacy levels. Incorporating multiple language options, culturally sensitive content, and simplifying complex medical jargon can enhance inclusivity and make these platforms more user-friendly for a wider audience.

Furthermore, internet-based health platforms should strive to be inclusive for individuals from different socioeconomic backgrounds. Access to affordable healthcare is a global concern, and internet-based platforms have the potential to bridge this gap by providing low-cost or free services. By offering affordable subscriptions, telemedicine consultations, or access to online health communities, these platforms can ensure that healthcare is accessible to everyone, regardless of their financial circumstances.

In conclusion, accessibility and inclusivity should be at the forefront of the design and development of internet-based health platforms. By considering the needs of individuals with physical disabilities, diverse cultural backgrounds, and varying socioeconomic statuses, these platforms can truly revolutionize the way we access and engage with healthcare services. Ultimately, the goal should be to maximize the potential of internet-based health platforms to improve the well-being and quality of life for all individuals, regardless of their internet proficiency or niche.

Overcoming Barriers to Adoption

In today's digital age, the internet plays a crucial role in various aspects of our lives, including healthcare. Internet-based health platforms have revolutionized the way we access and manage our health information, providing a convenient and efficient means of monitoring and improving our well-being. However, despite the numerous benefits offered by these platforms, there are still barriers that prevent widespread adoption. This subchapter aims to address these barriers and provide solutions for individuals to embrace the digital wellness revolution.

One significant barrier to adoption is the lack of digital literacy among individuals. Many people, particularly older adults, may feel overwhelmed or intimidated by technology. To overcome this barrier, it is crucial to provide comprehensive digital literacy programs that teach individuals how to navigate and utilize internet-based health platforms effectively. By empowering individuals with the necessary skills and knowledge, we can bridge the digital divide and ensure that everyone can benefit from these platforms.

Another barrier is the concern for privacy and security. With the increasing number of data breaches and online scams, individuals are rightfully cautious when it comes to sharing personal health information online. To address this, internet-based health platforms must prioritize data security and transparency. Implementing robust encryption measures, obtaining user consent, and providing clear privacy policies can help build trust and alleviate concerns. Educating individuals about the security measures in place and how their data is protected can also help overcome this barrier.

Limited access to high-speed internet is yet another obstacle to adoption. While internet connectivity has significantly improved over the years, there are still areas with inadequate infrastructure, particularly in rural or remote regions. To overcome this barrier, governments and organizations must invest in expanding broadband access to ensure that everyone has equal opportunities to utilize internet-based health platforms. Additionally, creating mobile-friendly applications that can function on slower internet connections can also help increase access.

Lastly, the lack of awareness and understanding about the benefits of internet-based health platforms can hinder adoption. Many individuals may not be aware of the vast array of resources available online or may not fully comprehend how these platforms can improve their overall well-being. To overcome this barrier, educational campaigns and initiatives should be launched to raise awareness about the advantages of these platforms. By showcasing real-life success stories and highlighting the impact of internet-based health platforms on individuals' lives, we can inspire more people to embrace this digital revolution.

In conclusion, while there are barriers to adoption, it is essential to overcome these obstacles to ensure that internet-based health platforms are accessible to everyone. By addressing digital literacy, privacy concerns, limited access to internet, and lack of awareness, we can maximize the potential of these platforms and empower individuals to take control of their health in the digital era. The digital wellness revolution is within our reach, and by working together, we can make it a reality for all.

In today's digital age, the internet has become an integral part of our lives, transforming the way we connect, communicate, and access information. One of the most significant advancements in this realm is the emergence of internet-based health platforms, which have the potential to revolutionize the healthcare industry. However, despite the numerous benefits and possibilities these platforms offer, there are still several barriers that hinder their widespread adoption. In this subchapter, we will explore some of these barriers and provide insights on how to overcome them, empowering individuals to embrace the digital wellness revolution.

One of the primary obstacles to adopting internet-based health platforms is the lack of awareness and understanding among the general public. Many individuals are unaware of the existence and potential benefits of these platforms, which leads to hesitancy and resistance. To overcome this barrier, it is crucial to educate and raise awareness among the masses. This can be done through various channels, such as public campaigns, community events, and partnerships with healthcare providers and organizations. By showcasing the transformative power of these platforms and their ability to improve health outcomes, we can engage and motivate individuals to embrace digital wellness.

Another significant barrier is the digital divide, which refers to the unequal access to technology and the internet. While the majority of the population may have access to the internet, there are still marginalized communities and individuals who face limited or no connectivity. To address this barrier, it is essential to bridge the digital divide by advocating for universal internet access and providing resources to underserved communities. This can be achieved through government initiatives, partnerships with technology companies, and community-driven efforts to establish internet infrastructure in remote areas. By ensuring equal access, we can empower everyone to benefit from internet-based health platforms.

Additionally, concerns about privacy and security pose a significant barrier to adoption. Many individuals worry about the confidentiality of their personal health information and the potential misuse of data. To address these concerns, it is crucial to establish robust data protection policies and regulations. Transparency and trust-building measures should be implemented by health platforms to assure users that their information is secure and will only be used for the intended purposes. Educating users about the privacy features and encryption protocols employed by these platforms can also alleviate concerns and encourage adoption.

In conclusion, while internet-based health platforms hold immense potential, overcoming barriers to adoption is crucial to ensure their widespread utilization. By raising awareness, bridging the digital divide, and addressing privacy concerns, we can empower individuals from all walks of life to embrace the digital wellness revolution. By working collectively to overcome these barriers, we can maximize the benefits of internet-based health platforms and create a healthier and more connected society for all.

In today's digital era, the internet has become an integral part of our lives, offering a multitude of health platforms that can revolutionize the way we approach wellness. However, despite the numerous benefits, there are still several barriers that hinder the widespread adoption of these internet-based health platforms. This subchapter aims to address these barriers and provide insights on how we can overcome them to fully embrace the digital wellness revolution.

One of the primary barriers to adoption is the lack of awareness and understanding of internet-based health platforms. Many individuals are unaware of the potential benefits these platforms offer, or they may have misconceptions about their effectiveness and reliability. To overcome this barrier, it is crucial to educate the general public about the capabilities and advantages of these platforms. By providing accessible and reliable information through various channels, such as online resources, social media campaigns, and community engagement, we can bridge the knowledge gap and ensure that everyone is well-informed about the potential of internet-based health platforms.

Another significant barrier is the digital divide, which refers to the unequal access to technology and the internet across different populations. While internet penetration has increased globally, certain communities, especially those in remote or underserved areas, still face limited access to reliable internet connections and affordable devices. To address this barrier, efforts must be made to bridge the digital divide by improving infrastructure, increasing affordability, and promoting digital literacy. Collaborations between governments, private organizations, and internet service providers can play a vital role in ensuring that internet-based health platforms are accessible to all, regardless of their geographical location or socioeconomic status.

Privacy and security concerns also act as barriers to adoption. Many individuals are hesitant to share personal health information online due to fears of data breaches and misuse of sensitive data. To overcome this barrier, stringent privacy regulations and security measures must be put in place to safeguard user data. Transparent communication about how data is collected, stored, and used can help build trust and alleviate concerns. Additionally, educating individuals about the benefits of sharing their health information can help them make informed decisions and embrace the potential of internet-based health platforms.

In conclusion, while there are barriers to the widespread adoption of internet-based health platforms, they can be overcome through education, bridging the digital divide, and ensuring privacy and security. By addressing these barriers, we can empower individuals from all walks of life to embrace the digital wellness revolution and harness the power of the internet to optimize their health and well-being. It is up to all of us, as a society, to work together and ensure that no one is left behind in this transformative journey towards a healthier and more connected future.

Chapter 6: The Future of Internet-based Health Platforms

Innovations and Advancements

The world of internet-based health platforms is constantly evolving, with new innovations and advancements emerging every day. In this subchapter, we will explore the latest breakthroughs in technology and how they are revolutionizing digital wellness for everyone.

One of the most significant innovations in recent years is the rise of wearable devices. These smart gadgets, such as fitness trackers and smartwatches, have become increasingly popular among individuals seeking to improve their health and well-being. With the ability to monitor heart rate, track physical activity, and provide personalized feedback, wearables have empowered individuals to take control of their own health like never before. Whether you are an athlete looking to optimize performance or simply someone trying to stay active, these devices offer valuable insights and motivation.

Another exciting advancement in internet-based health platforms is the integration of artificial intelligence (AI) and machine learning. These technologies have the potential to transform the way we approach healthcare by analyzing vast amounts of data and providing personalized recommendations. AI-powered chatbots, for example, can offer immediate support and guidance, answering common health-related questions and even providing mental health support. Furthermore, machine learning algorithms can identify patterns in data to predict and prevent potential health issues, allowing individuals to proactively manage their well-being.

Additionally, virtual reality (VR) and augmented reality (AR) have emerged as powerful tools in the digital wellness revolution. VR technology immerses users in simulated environments, offering unique opportunities for therapeutic interventions, such as pain management and exposure therapy. AR, on the other hand, overlays digital information onto the real world, providing valuable visual cues and guidance. From helping individuals visualize their fitness goals to assisting healthcare professionals in complex surgical procedures, these immersive technologies have endless applications in the realm of health and wellness.

Lastly, advancements in telemedicine have greatly expanded access to healthcare services. Through internet-based platforms, individuals can now consult with healthcare providers remotely, eliminating the need for in-person visits and reducing barriers to care. This is particularly beneficial for individuals in underserved areas or those with mobility constraints. Telemedicine has also played a crucial role in managing the ongoing COVID-19 pandemic, allowing individuals to receive medical advice and prescriptions from the safety of their homes.

In conclusion, the innovations and advancements in internet-based health platforms have transformed the way we approach wellness. From wearable devices and AI-powered chatbots to VR and telemedicine, these technologies have empowered individuals to take control of their health and well-being like never before. As the digital wellness revolution continues to unfold, we can expect even more exciting developments on the horizon, providing greater access, convenience, and personalized care for everyone.

In today's fast-paced digital age, the internet has revolutionized almost every aspect of our lives, including the way we approach health and wellness. The internet has become a powerful tool in enhancing our well-being, connecting us to a world of information, resources, and communities dedicated to improving our overall health. This subchapter explores the innovations and advancements in internet-based health platforms that have shaped the digital wellness revolution.

One of the most significant advancements in internet-based health platforms is the rise of telemedicine. With the ability to consult with healthcare professionals remotely, patients can now receive medical advice, diagnosis, and even treatment from the comfort of their own homes. Telemedicine has not only made healthcare more accessible but has also allowed for timely interventions, especially in rural or underserved areas. This innovation has transformed the way we approach healthcare, ensuring that individuals can receive the care they need, regardless of their location.

Another innovation that has gained tremendous popularity is the use of health and wellness apps. These apps offer a wide range of features, from tracking physical activity and nutrition to providing guided meditation and sleep monitoring. These apps empower individuals to take control of their health, providing them with personalized insights and recommendations. With the help of these apps, users can set goals, track progress, and make informed decisions about their well-being, all within the convenience of their smartphones.

Furthermore, the internet has fostered the growth of online communities and support networks focused on specific health conditions or wellness goals. These communities provide a safe and inclusive space for individuals to share their experiences, seek advice, and find support from like-minded individuals. The power of these communities lies in their ability to connect individuals who may feel isolated or misunderstood, allowing them to find solace and strength in their shared struggles and triumphs.

Lastly, the internet has revolutionized the way healthcare professionals collaborate and share knowledge. Online platforms enable healthcare providers to connect, exchange best practices, and access the latest research and advancements in their respective fields. This interconnectedness allows for greater collaboration, ultimately leading to improved patient care and outcomes.

The innovations and advancements in internet-based health platforms have undoubtedly transformed the way we approach our well-being. From telemedicine to health apps and online communities, the digital wellness revolution has empowered individuals to take control of their health, connect with others, and access resources that were once out of reach. It is an exciting time for the internet and the world of health, as we continue to witness the limitless potential of these innovations in enhancing our overall well-being.

The internet has revolutionized numerous aspects of our lives, and the field of health is no exception. In recent years, we have witnessed remarkable innovations and advancements in internet-based health platforms that have transformed the way we approach wellness. This subchapter explores some of the most groundbreaking developments in this field, highlighting their potential to improve the health and well-being of individuals from all walks of life.

One of the most significant advancements in internet-based health platforms is the rise of telemedicine. With the power of the internet, individuals can now connect with healthcare professionals remotely, eliminating the need for physical visits to clinics or hospitals. Telemedicine has proven particularly beneficial for those living in remote areas or with limited mobility, as it allows them to access quality healthcare services from the comfort of their own homes. Moreover, telemedicine has played a crucial role in improving healthcare accessibility during the ongoing COVID-19 pandemic, ensuring that individuals can receive medical attention without risking exposure to the virus.

Another area of innovation in internet-based health platforms is the development of wearable technology. From fitness trackers to smartwatches, these devices have revolutionized the way we monitor our health and fitness levels. Wearables can track various metrics such as heart rate, sleep patterns, and physical activity, providing individuals with valuable insights into their overall well-being. These devices often sync with mobile applications or online platforms, allowing users to analyze their data and set personalized health goals. The availability of real-time health data has empowered individuals to take control of their own health and make informed decisions about their lifestyle choices.

Furthermore, the advent of artificial intelligence (AI) has opened up new possibilities in the realm of internet-based health platforms. AI algorithms can analyze vast amounts of medical data, aiding in the diagnosis and treatment of various conditions. Additionally, AI-powered chatbots and virtual assistants offer personalized health advice and support, enhancing the accessibility and affordability of healthcare services.

As the internet continues to evolve, so do the innovations and advancements in internet-based health platforms. These developments have the potential to transform healthcare delivery, making it more efficient, accessible, and patient-centered. By harnessing the power of the internet, individuals can take charge of their own health, connect with healthcare professionals remotely, and benefit from personalized insights and support. The digital wellness revolution is well underway, and it is set to redefine the future of healthcare for everyone, regardless of their internet proficiency.

Artificial Intelligence in Health Platforms

In recent years, the rapid advancements in technology, particularly in the field of Artificial Intelligence (AI), have revolutionized various industries, and the healthcare sector is no exception. AI has emerged as a game-changer, transforming the way we approach healthcare and enabling the development of powerful digital platforms that have the potential to maximize our well-being. In this subchapter, we will explore the fascinating world of Artificial Intelligence in Health Platforms.

Internet-based health platforms have become increasingly popular, offering a wide range of services and resources to individuals seeking to improve their well-being. These platforms leverage AI technology to provide personalized and targeted solutions, making them invaluable tools in the digital wellness revolution.

One of the key benefits of AI in health platforms is its ability to analyze vast amounts of data quickly and accurately. By harnessing machine learning algorithms, these platforms can process and interpret medical records, research papers, and other relevant information to generate insights and recommendations. This not only saves time for healthcare professionals but also allows for better diagnoses, treatment plans, and preventative measures.

AI-powered health platforms also excel in providing personalized recommendations based on individual health data and preferences. By collecting and analyzing data such as medical history, fitness levels, and lifestyle choices, these platforms can offer tailored advice on nutrition, exercise, sleep patterns, and stress management. This personalized approach enhances user engagement and motivation, leading to better health outcomes.

Furthermore, AI can play a crucial role in patient monitoring and early detection of health issues. Through wearable devices and sensors, health platforms can continuously monitor vital signs, alerting users and healthcare providers to any abnormalities or potential risks. This real-time monitoring can prevent emergencies, detect diseases at early stages, and enable timely interventions.

Another exciting application of AI in health platforms is virtual assistants and chatbots. These intelligent agents can provide immediate responses to user inquiries, offering medical advice, appointment scheduling, and even mental health support. Virtual assistants are available 24/7, eliminating the need to wait for a healthcare professional's availability and increasing accessibility to healthcare services.

In conclusion, the integration of Artificial Intelligence in health platforms has opened up tremendous possibilities for enhancing our well-being in the digital age. These platforms empower individuals to take control of their health, providing personalized recommendations, real-time monitoring, and immediate access to medical advice. As the digital wellness revolution continues to unfold, AI will undoubtedly remain at the forefront of innovation in the interplay between the internet and healthcare.

Artificial Intelligence (AI) has revolutionized various industries, and the healthcare sector is no exception. As the world becomes increasingly digital, the integration of AI into health platforms has paved the way for a new era of personalized and efficient healthcare services. In this subchapter, we will explore the transformative power of AI in health platforms and its impact on the internet-based wellness revolution.

AI, in its simplest terms, refers to the ability of machines to mimic human intelligence and perform tasks that typically require human intelligence. In the context of health platforms, AI algorithms are used to analyze vast amounts of data, identify patterns, and make predictions. This enables healthcare providers to offer individualized care, improve diagnosis accuracy, and streamline treatment plans.

One of the key benefits of incorporating AI into health platforms is the ability to process and analyze large datasets quickly. This allows healthcare providers to leverage data from electronic health records, wearable devices, and other sources to gain insights into patient health trends and make informed decisions. AI algorithms can identify patterns that might not be apparent to human physicians, aiding in early detection of diseases and improving overall patient outcomes.

Moreover, AI-powered chatbots and virtual assistants have become increasingly prevalent in health platforms. These tools provide users with round-the-clock access to medical information, personalized recommendations, and even basic diagnostic assistance. By leveraging AI, health platforms can offer immediate support and guidance to users, reducing the burden on healthcare systems and empowering individuals to take charge of their own health.

Another noteworthy application of AI in health platforms is in the field of precision medicine. AI algorithms can analyze genetic data, medical records, and clinical research to identify personalized treatment plans for individuals. This approach has the potential to revolutionize disease management by tailoring treatments to a patient's unique genetic makeup and medical history, maximizing efficacy and minimizing side effects.

However, as with any emerging technology, there are challenges and ethical considerations that need to be addressed. Privacy concerns, data security, and the potential for bias in AI algorithms are important areas that require ongoing attention and regulation.

In conclusion, the integration of AI into health platforms is transforming the way healthcare is delivered and experienced. The internet-based wellness revolution is empowered by AI's ability to process vast amounts of data, provide personalized recommendations, and improve diagnosis accuracy. As this technology continues to evolve, it holds tremendous potential for improving healthcare outcomes and empowering individuals to lead healthier lives.

The integration of artificial intelligence (AI) into health platforms has heralded a new era in healthcare. With the advent of the digital revolution, the internet has become an integral part of our lives, and its potential in the field of healthcare is vast. This subchapter explores the power of AI in health platforms and how it is revolutionizing the way we approach our well-being.

AI technology has rapidly advanced in recent years, enabling health platforms to provide personalized and efficient care to individuals across the globe. By leveraging vast amounts of data, AI algorithms can analyze and interpret medical information more accurately than ever before. This allows healthcare professionals to make more informed decisions and provide tailored treatment plans to patients.

One of the key advantages of AI in health platforms is its ability to assist in early disease detection. With AI-powered diagnostic tools, medical professionals can detect diseases at their earliest stages, leading to more successful treatment outcomes. These tools can analyze medical images, such as X-rays and MRIs, with incredible precision, helping doctors identify abnormalities that may have previously gone unnoticed.

Moreover, AI in health platforms enables the development of virtual assistants and chatbots that can provide medical advice and support around the clock. These AI-powered assistants can answer questions, provide accurate information, and even triage patients based on their symptoms. This not only improves accessibility to healthcare but also reduces the burden on healthcare systems, allowing medical professionals to focus on more critical cases.

Another area where AI excels is in predictive analytics. By analyzing vast amounts of patient data, AI algorithms can identify patterns and predict potential health risks. This proactive approach allows healthcare providers to intervene before a condition worsens, reducing hospitalizations and improving overall health outcomes.

However, it is crucial to address the ethical and security concerns surrounding AI in health platforms. Privacy and data protection must be a top priority to ensure that patient information remains confidential and secure. Additionally, the potential for bias in AI algorithms must be carefully monitored to ensure fair and equitable healthcare.

In conclusion, the integration of AI into health platforms has transformed the way we approach healthcare. Through early disease detection, virtual assistants, and predictive analytics, AI is revolutionizing the field and maximizing the potential of internet-based health platforms. As we continue to harness the power of AI, it is essential to prioritize privacy, security, and ethical considerations to ensure that these technologies benefit everyone and contribute to a healthier future.

Virtual Reality and Augmented Reality Applications

Virtual Reality (VR) and Augmented Reality (AR) have revolutionized the way we experience the digital world. These cutting-edge technologies have found applications in various fields, including entertainment, education, healthcare, and even e-commerce. In this subchapter, we will explore the incredible potential of VR and AR applications, specifically in the context of the internet.

One of the most significant areas where VR and AR have made a massive impact is in the field of entertainment. With VR headsets, users can immerse themselves in virtual worlds, experiencing games, movies, and even live events in a way that was previously unimaginable. AR, on the other hand, overlays digital information onto the real world, allowing users to interact with virtual objects and characters in their immediate surroundings. Both technologies have opened up new possibilities for interactive storytelling and have completely transformed the way we consume content online.

Education is another niche that has greatly benefited from VR and AR applications. Traditional learning methods can sometimes be limited in their ability to engage students. However, with VR and AR, students can explore historical landmarks, travel to distant galaxies, or dissect virtual organisms, all from the comfort of their classrooms. These technologies have the potential to make learning more interactive, engaging, and memorable, thereby enhancing the educational experience for learners of all ages.

In the realm of healthcare, VR and AR have proven to be invaluable tools. VR simulations can be used for medical training, allowing students and professionals to practice surgeries or complex medical procedures in a risk-free environment. AR applications can assist surgeons during operations, providing real-time information and guidance. Additionally, VR has shown promise in pain management by creating immersive experiences that distract patients from their discomfort.

E-commerce has also embraced VR and AR technologies, enhancing the online shopping experience. With VR, customers can virtually try on clothes, visualize furniture in their homes, or even test drive cars, all without leaving their living rooms. AR, on the other hand, allows users to scan products and view additional information or reviews in real-time, enhancing their purchasing decisions.

In conclusion, VR and AR have revolutionized the internet by offering immersive and interactive experiences across various niches. Whether it is for entertainment, education, healthcare, or e-commerce, these technologies have the potential to transform the way we engage with digital content. As they continue to evolve, VR and AR applications will undoubtedly shape the future of the internet and provide exciting opportunities for users of all backgrounds.

Virtual Reality (VR) and Augmented Reality (AR) have revolutionized the way we interact with technology and have opened up new possibilities in various fields. From gaming to education and healthcare, VR and AR applications have transformed the internet landscape, providing immersive experiences and enhancing user engagement.

In the realm of gaming, VR has taken players into a whole new dimension, allowing them to step inside their favorite virtual worlds. With a VR headset and motion controllers, gamers can now physically interact with their surroundings, making the gaming experience more realistic and captivating than ever before. AR, on the other hand, blends the virtual world with the real world, enhancing gameplay by overlaying digital elements onto the user's physical environment. This technology has given rise to popular games like Pokémon Go, where players can explore the real world while catching virtual creatures.

Beyond gaming, VR and AR have found applications in education and training. Virtual reality simulations can recreate historical events, scientific experiments, or even geographical locations, providing students with an immersive and interactive learning experience. AR, on the other hand, can enhance traditional textbooks by overlaying additional information, animations, and 3D models onto the pages, making learning more engaging and memorable.

In the healthcare industry, VR and AR have proven to be valuable tools. Surgeons can use VR simulations to practice complex procedures before performing them on real patients, reducing the risk of errors and improving overall surgical outcomes. AR can assist doctors during surgeries by overlaying patient data and medical images onto their field of view, providing real-time information without the need to divert their attention from the operation.

Moreover, VR has also been used to treat various psychological conditions, such as anxiety disorders and phobias. By creating virtual environments that trigger specific fears or anxieties, therapists can guide patients through exposure therapy in a controlled and safe manner.

In conclusion, VR and AR technologies have revolutionized the internet landscape, offering immersive and engaging experiences across various fields. From gaming and education to healthcare, these applications have transformed the way we interact with technology, opening up new possibilities and improving outcomes. As the technology continues to advance, the potential for VR and AR to shape the future of the internet remains vast, promising even more exciting and innovative applications for everyone to enjoy.

In today's digital age, the internet has revolutionized various aspects of our lives, including the field of healthcare. With the development of innovative technologies such as virtual reality (VR) and augmented reality (AR), the possibilities for improving our well-being and accessing healthcare services have expanded significantly.

VR and AR applications have gained popularity across different niches, and the internet serves as a platform for their widespread availability. These technologies provide immersive experiences that can enhance our understanding of health-related topics and improve the delivery of healthcare services.

One of the key applications of VR in the healthcare industry is medical training and education. Through virtual simulations, medical professionals can practice complex procedures and gain hands-on experience in a safe and controlled environment. This helps to improve their skills and reduce the risk of errors during real-life surgeries or treatments. Additionally, VR enables medical students to explore the human body in a three-dimensional space, enhancing their learning and comprehension of anatomical structures.

Another significant application of VR and AR is in mental health therapy. By creating virtual environments, individuals can confront their fears and anxieties in a controlled setting, aiding in the treatment of phobias, post-traumatic stress disorder (PTSD), and other psychological conditions. These immersive experiences, combined with therapeutic techniques, provide a powerful tool for mental health professionals to deliver effective treatment remotely through the internet.

In the realm of patient care, VR and AR have the potential to transform the way we receive medical services. Telemedicine platforms utilizing these technologies allow patients to consult with healthcare providers remotely, reducing the need for physical visits to clinics or hospitals. This not only saves time and money but also improves access to healthcare services, particularly for individuals living in remote areas or those with limited mobility.

Furthermore, VR and AR can be utilized for pain management. By immersing patients in virtual environments or overlaying digital elements onto the real world, these technologies can distract individuals from their pain, reducing the need for medication and enhancing overall well-being.

In conclusion, the internet has become a pivotal platform for the integration of VR and AR applications in healthcare. These technologies provide immense potential for medical training, mental health therapy, patient care, and pain management. As the digital wellness revolution continues to unfold, the internet will play a crucial role in maximizing the benefits of VR and AR in improving our overall health and well-being.

Ethical Considerations in Digital Health

In today's digital age, the internet has revolutionized various aspects of our lives, including healthcare. The emergence of digital health platforms has provided individuals with unprecedented access to information, resources, and services. However, it is crucial to navigate this digital wellness revolution with careful ethical considerations.

One of the primary ethical concerns in digital health is the privacy and security of personal health information. As we increasingly rely on internet-based health platforms, we are entrusting our sensitive data to these platforms. It is important to ensure that these platforms have robust security measures in place to protect our information from unauthorized access or breaches. Additionally, users should be aware of the data collection practices of these platforms and how their information is being used.

Another ethical consideration is the potential for bias in digital health platforms. Algorithms and artificial intelligence play a significant role in analyzing vast amounts of data and providing personalized health recommendations. However, if these algorithms are biased or based on incomplete or inaccurate data, it could lead to discrimination or suboptimal care for certain individuals or communities. It is essential for developers and practitioners to continuously assess and mitigate any biases that may arise in these platforms.

Furthermore, digital health platforms must prioritize user consent and autonomy. Users should have the ability to control and manage their personal health information, including the choice to opt out of certain data collection or sharing practices. Clear and transparent consent processes should be implemented to ensure that users are fully informed about how their data will be used.

The accessibility and inclusivity of digital health platforms are also important ethical considerations. Internet-based health platforms should be designed to be accessible to individuals with disabilities, ensuring that they can fully benefit from these services. Moreover, efforts should be made to bridge the digital divide and ensure that internet access is available to underserved communities, as lack of access can exacerbate existing health disparities.

Lastly, ethical considerations in digital health extend to professional standards and accountability. Healthcare professionals who utilize digital health platforms must adhere to ethical guidelines and standards of practice. They should undergo proper training and education to ensure that they are competent in using these platforms and providing appropriate care.

In conclusion, as the digital wellness revolution continues to shape the healthcare landscape, ethical considerations are paramount. Privacy, bias, consent, accessibility, and professional accountability should all be addressed to maximize the potential benefits of internet-based health platforms. By embracing these ethical principles, we can build a digital health ecosystem that is inclusive, secure, and responsive to the needs of every individual.

In an era of rapid technological advancements, digital health has emerged as a game-changer in the healthcare industry. Internet-based health platforms have revolutionized the way we access and manage our health information, making healthcare more convenient and accessible. However, with this digital revolution comes a set of ethical considerations that need to be addressed to ensure the responsible and ethical use of these platforms.

One of the primary ethical concerns in digital health is the protection of personal health information. As we increasingly rely on internet-based platforms to store and share our health data, there is a need to ensure that this information remains confidential and secure. Healthcare providers and technology companies must invest in robust security measures to safeguard sensitive data from potential breaches or unauthorized access.

Furthermore, the issue of consent and privacy arises when it comes to the collection and use of personal health data. Users must have a clear understanding of how their data will be collected, stored, and used by these platforms. Transparent privacy policies and obtaining informed consent are crucial in maintaining trust between users and healthcare providers.

Another ethical consideration is the potential for bias and discrimination in digital health platforms. As these platforms use algorithms to analyze and interpret health data, there is a risk of perpetuating existing biases or discriminating against certain individuals or communities. Developers and researchers must be aware of these biases and work towards creating algorithms that are fair and unbiased.

Additionally, the digital divide is an ethical concern that needs to be addressed in the context of internet-based health platforms. While these platforms have the potential to improve access to healthcare, they may inadvertently exclude those who do not have access to the internet or lack digital literacy skills. Efforts should be made to bridge this gap and ensure that digital health platforms are accessible to all, regardless of socioeconomic status or geographical location.

Lastly, the issue of accountability and responsibility arises in digital health. Who is responsible if a digital health platform provides inaccurate or misleading information? Healthcare providers, technology companies, and regulatory bodies must establish clear guidelines and standards to ensure the accuracy and reliability of these platforms.

In conclusion, while internet-based health platforms offer numerous benefits, it is crucial to address the ethical considerations that accompany this digital revolution. Protecting personal health information, ensuring consent and privacy, mitigating bias and discrimination, bridging the digital divide, and establishing accountability are all essential aspects of ethical digital health practices. By addressing these considerations, we can maximize the potential of internet-based health platforms while ensuring the responsible and ethical use of technology in healthcare.

In today's digital age, the internet has revolutionized the way we live, work, and even how we manage our health. With the rise of internet-based health platforms, individuals now have access to a vast array of tools and resources to monitor and improve their well-being. However, this digital wellness revolution also brings forth a range of ethical considerations that must be carefully addressed.

One of the primary ethical concerns in the realm of digital health is the privacy and security of personal health information. As we increasingly rely on internet-based platforms to store and transmit sensitive data, such as medical records and health tracking data, it becomes crucial to prioritize robust security measures. This includes encryption, strict access controls, and regular audits to ensure that personal information remains confidential and protected from unauthorized access.

Moreover, the issue of informed consent is vital in the digital health landscape. Individuals must be fully aware of how their data will be collected, used, and shared by these platforms. Clear and transparent policies should be in place, outlining the purpose of data collection, potential risks, and the individual's rights regarding their personal information. This allows users to make informed decisions about participating in digital health platforms and ensures that their autonomy and privacy are respected.

Another ethical consideration is the potential for bias and discrimination in digital health tools and algorithms. As these platforms rely on data-driven insights to provide personalized recommendations and diagnoses, there is a risk that certain populations or individuals may be disproportionately affected. Developers and healthcare professionals must be vigilant in identifying and addressing these biases to ensure equal access and fair treatment for all users.

Furthermore, the accessibility of digital health platforms is a crucial ethical concern. While the internet has opened up vast opportunities for health management, it is essential to consider those individuals who may not have access to reliable internet connections or the necessary technical skills to navigate these platforms. Efforts should be made to bridge the digital divide and ensure that everyone, regardless of socioeconomic status or location, can benefit from digital health innovations.

In conclusion, the digital wellness revolution has undoubtedly transformed the healthcare landscape, providing individuals with unprecedented access to health information and resources. However, it is crucial to address the ethical considerations that arise in this digital age. Privacy, informed consent, bias, and accessibility are just a few of the ethical concerns that must be carefully navigated to ensure that the benefits of digital health are enjoyed by everyone, regardless of their internet niche. By prioritizing ethical considerations, we can create a digital health ecosystem that empowers individuals while upholding their rights and well-being.

Data Privacy and Consent

In this digital age, where the internet has become an integral part of our lives, ensuring data privacy and obtaining consent are critical aspects that cannot be overlooked. The vast amount of personal information shared online raises concerns about the security and protection of sensitive data. This subchapter delves into the importance of data privacy and consent in the realm of the internet and explores the measures individuals can take to safeguard their information.

Data privacy refers to the control individuals have over their personal data and how it is collected, used, and shared by organizations. It encompasses the right to know what information is being collected, the purpose for which it is being used, and the ability to grant or revoke consent. With the proliferation of internet-based health platforms, the collection of personal health data has become more prevalent. Understanding and managing data privacy are paramount when it comes to maintaining the trust and confidence of users.

Consent, on the other hand, is the explicit permission given by individuals for their data to be used for specific purposes. It is crucial that consent is informed and freely given, without any coercion or hidden agenda. Consent should be sought in a clear and easily understandable manner, ensuring that individuals are aware of the data being collected and how it will be used. Furthermore, users should be empowered to withdraw their consent at any point in time.

To protect data privacy and ensure consent, individuals must take an active role in managing their online presence. This includes being cautious about the information shared on social media platforms, using strong and unique passwords, and being mindful of the permissions granted to applications and websites. Regularly reviewing privacy settings and considering the use of privacy-enhancing tools can also enhance data protection.

Organizations also have a responsibility to prioritize data privacy and consent. They should implement robust security measures, such as encryption and secure storage, to safeguard user data. Transparency in data handling practices and obtaining explicit consent should be integral to their operations. Additionally, organizations should educate users about their rights and provide clear avenues for addressing privacy concerns.

In conclusion, data privacy and consent are indispensable in the world of the internet. As individuals become more reliant on internet-based health platforms, it is crucial to be vigilant about protecting personal data. By understanding the importance of data privacy, actively managing online presence, and demanding transparency and consent from organizations, we can collectively ensure a safer and more secure digital environment.

In this digital age, where the internet has become an integral part of our lives, it is crucial to understand the importance of data privacy and consent. The vast amount of personal information that we share online has raised concerns about how it is collected, stored, and used by various internet platforms. This subchapter aims to shed light on the significance of data privacy and the role of consent in maintaining a safe and secure online experience.

Data privacy refers to the protection of personal information from unauthorized access, use, or disclosure. With the internet being a treasure trove of data, it is essential to safeguard our personal information, including our health data, from falling into the wrong hands. Internet-based health platforms, in particular, handle sensitive data related to our well-being, making data privacy even more critical.

One of the primary ways to protect our data is by being aware of the privacy policies and terms of service of the platforms we use. These documents outline how our data will be collected, stored, and used. Understanding these policies empowers us to make informed decisions about the platforms we choose to engage with.

Equally important is obtaining consent before sharing any personal information. Consent plays a crucial role in ensuring that our data is used only for the purposes we intend. Internet platforms should provide clear and transparent explanations about how our data will be utilized and seek our consent before collecting or sharing it. As users, we have the right to control how our data is used and should be able to revoke consent at any time.

To protect our data privacy, it is advisable to use strong and unique passwords for online accounts, enable two-factor authentication whenever possible, and regularly review privacy settings. Additionally, being cautious while sharing personal information on social media and avoiding suspicious websites can further enhance our online safety.

In conclusion, data privacy and consent are paramount in the digital wellness revolution. As internet users, we must be vigilant about our personal information and take necessary steps to protect it. By understanding privacy policies, giving informed consent, and adopting secure online practices, we can ensure a safer and more secure internet experience for ourselves and others. Together, we can embrace the digital world while safeguarding our privacy.

In today's digital age, where internet usage has become an integral part of our lives, it is crucial to address the issue of data privacy and consent. With the rapid advancement of technology and the increasing popularity of internet-based health platforms, it is essential for everyone to understand the importance of safeguarding their personal information.

The concept of data privacy refers to the protection of an individual's personal data from unauthorized access or use. In the context of internet-based health platforms, this includes sensitive information such as medical records, health conditions, and other personal details. It is vital for users to be aware of how their data is collected, stored, and used by these platforms.

Consent plays a significant role in data privacy. Informed consent means that individuals have a clear understanding of how their personal data will be utilized and have given their explicit permission for its use. Internet-based health platforms should prioritize obtaining consent from users before collecting any personal information, ensuring transparency in their data collection practices.

To protect your data privacy and give informed consent, there are a few key steps to follow. First and foremost, always read the platform's privacy policy and terms of service. These documents outline how your data will be handled and shared. Look for platforms that have stringent security measures in place, such as encryption and secure servers, to protect your information from unauthorized access.

Another important aspect to consider is the sharing of your data. Understand which parties have access to your information and for what purpose. If a platform shares your data with third parties, make sure they have strict data protection policies in place.

It is also crucial to be mindful of your own actions online. Avoid sharing sensitive personal information on public forums or social media platforms, as this can increase the risk of unauthorized access. Be cautious when downloading apps or granting permissions on your devices, as some may collect more data than necessary.

Ultimately, data privacy and consent are everyone's responsibility. By being informed, proactive, and vigilant about how our personal information is handled, we can ensure our digital wellness and protect ourselves from potential risks.

Ensuring Ethical Use of AI and Personalization

In today's digital age, the internet has become an integral part of our lives. It has revolutionized the way we access information, communicate, and even manage our health. Internet-based health platforms and Artificial Intelligence (AI) have emerged as powerful tools that can greatly enhance our well-being. However, with this power comes the responsibility to ensure ethical use of AI and personalization in the internet realm.

AI has the potential to transform healthcare by providing personalized recommendations, diagnosing diseases, and even predicting health risks. However, the use of AI in healthcare raises several ethical concerns that need to be addressed. One major concern is privacy. With the vast amount of personal data being collected, it is crucial to have strict regulations in place to protect individuals' privacy. Healthcare platforms must ensure that personal information is secure and only used for the intended purpose.

Transparency is another key aspect of ensuring ethical use of AI. Users should be informed about how their data is being collected, stored, and used. Clear guidelines and consent mechanisms should be in place to ensure individuals are aware of the data being collected and have control over its usage. It is important to foster a culture of transparency and accountability among internet-based health platforms to build trust with users.

Bias is another ethical concern in AI and personalization. AI algorithms are trained on large datasets, and if these datasets are biased, it can lead to biased outcomes. Developers must ensure that their algorithms are trained on diverse datasets that represent the population accurately. Regular audits and evaluations should be conducted to identify and mitigate any biases in the AI system.

Moreover, the internet-based health platforms should prioritize the well-being of their users over profit. They should ensure that the recommendations and personalized content they provide are evidence-based and reliable. Misleading or inaccurate information can have serious consequences for users' health.

To address these ethical concerns, collaboration between internet-based health platforms, regulators, and healthcare professionals is crucial. A multidisciplinary approach is needed to develop ethical frameworks and guidelines for the use of AI and personalization in healthcare. Additionally, ongoing research and evaluation are necessary to keep up with the evolving landscape of technology and healthcare.

In conclusion, the ethical use of AI and personalization in internet-based health platforms is essential to maximize their potential for improving well-being. Privacy, transparency, bias, and user well-being should be at the forefront of considerations. By addressing these concerns and fostering collaboration, we can ensure that the digital wellness revolution truly benefits everyone and creates a healthier future.

In today's digital era, we are witnessing the rapid growth and integration of artificial intelligence (AI) and personalization in various aspects of our lives, especially on the Internet. As these technologies become increasingly prevalent, it is crucial to address the ethical considerations surrounding their use. This subchapter aims to shed light on the importance of ensuring ethical practices in the realm of AI and personalization, particularly within the internet niche.

First and foremost, it is essential to understand the potential impact of AI and personalization on individuals' privacy and data security. With the vast amount of personal information available online, there is a pressing need to establish strict guidelines and regulations to protect users from unauthorized data access or misuse. Internet platforms must prioritize user consent and transparency, ensuring that individuals have control over the data they share and are aware of how it will be used.

Furthermore, ethical considerations extend beyond privacy concerns. AI algorithms and personalized recommendations have the power to shape individuals' online experiences, influencing their decisions and beliefs. This raises questions about the potential manipulation or bias that can arise from such technologies. To mitigate these risks, internet platforms should implement robust safeguards to ensure fairness, transparency, and accountability in the algorithms they employ.

Another critical aspect of ethical AI and personalization is the potential for discrimination and exclusion. If these technologies are not carefully designed and tested, they may inadvertently perpetuate existing biases or create new ones. For example, biased algorithms in healthcare platforms might lead to unequal access to medical resources or treatments. To address this, developers and policymakers must actively work towards inclusivity, diversity, and fairness in the development and deployment of AI and personalization technologies.

Ultimately, ensuring ethical use of AI and personalization requires collaboration between internet platforms, regulators, and users themselves. Platforms must adopt ethical frameworks and codes of conduct, while regulators must establish clear guidelines to govern their use. Users, on the other hand, must be actively engaged in understanding and advocating for their rights and interests in the digital world.

By prioritizing ethics in the use of AI and personalization, we can harness the full potential of these technologies while safeguarding privacy, promoting fairness, and fostering inclusivity. It is crucial that all stakeholders come together to address these ethical challenges and work towards a digital environment that maximizes the benefits of internet-based health platforms while minimizing the risks. Only then can we truly revolutionize digital wellness and create a more equitable and empowering online experience for everyone.

In the digital age, the internet has become an integral part of our lives, transforming the way we access information, communicate, and even manage our health. With the advent of artificial intelligence (AI) and personalization algorithms, the internet has the potential to revolutionize the way we receive health-related services and information. However, as we embrace these advancements, it is crucial to ensure their ethical use.

AI algorithms have the power to provide personalized health recommendations, tailored treatment plans, and even predict potential health risks. This technology has the ability to significantly improve healthcare outcomes and empower individuals to take charge of their well-being. However, there are concerns surrounding the privacy, security, and biases associated with AI algorithms.

Privacy and security are paramount when it comes to utilizing AI and personalization technologies. As individuals entrust their personal health information to internet-based platforms, it is essential that stringent measures are in place to safeguard this data. Internet platforms must adhere to robust data protection protocols, ensuring that personal information is encrypted, stored securely, and accessible only to authorized individuals. Transparency is also crucial, as users need to know how their data is being used and have the option to opt out if they so choose.

Another important consideration is the potential for biases within AI algorithms. These algorithms learn from historical data, and if this data is biased, it can perpetuate inequalities in healthcare. Efforts should be made to ensure that AI algorithms are built on diverse datasets that represent the entire population, rather than perpetuating existing biases. Regular audits and evaluations should be conducted to detect and rectify any biases that may arise.

Furthermore, it is essential to strike a balance between personalization and autonomy. While personalized recommendations can be highly beneficial, individuals should have the freedom to make their own choices regarding their health. Internet-based platforms must provide users with accurate, evidence-based information and empower them to make informed decisions.

In conclusion, the ethical use of AI and personalization in internet-based health platforms is crucial to ensure the well-being of individuals. Privacy, security, and the prevention of biases should be prioritized to build trust and confidence in these technologies. By embracing ethical practices and striving for inclusivity, we can maximize the potential of the digital wellness revolution and create a healthier future for all.

The Potential Impact on Healthcare Systems

In this digital age, the internet has become an integral part of our lives, revolutionizing the way we connect, communicate, and access information. The impact of the internet on various industries, including healthcare, has been immense. As we delve into the potential impact on healthcare systems, it becomes evident that the internet has the power to transform the way we approach healthcare, making it more accessible, efficient, and patient-centric.

One of the most significant impacts of the internet on healthcare systems is the democratization of information. The internet has empowered individuals to access a wealth of health-related information, allowing them to become active participants in their own well-being. With a simple search query, anyone can find information about symptoms, treatment options, and preventive measures for various health conditions. This newfound knowledge enables individuals to make informed decisions about their health, leading to improved outcomes and reduced reliance on healthcare professionals for every minor concern.

Internet-based health platforms have also revolutionized the way healthcare is delivered, making it more convenient and accessible. Telemedicine, for example, has emerged as a game-changer, allowing patients to consult with healthcare professionals remotely, eliminating the need for physical visits to clinics or hospitals. This is particularly beneficial for individuals living in remote areas with limited access to healthcare facilities. Furthermore, telemedicine reduces the burden on healthcare systems, minimizing waiting times and allowing healthcare professionals to focus on more critical cases.

The internet has also paved the way for the development of innovative healthcare technologies and solutions. From wearable devices that monitor vital signs in real-time to mobile applications that track and manage chronic conditions, these technologies have the potential to revolutionize healthcare delivery. The integration of these technologies with internet-based platforms enables healthcare professionals to collect and analyze vast amounts of patient data, facilitating personalized and proactive care.

However, while the potential impact of the internet on healthcare systems is immense, it is essential to address the challenges that come with it. Privacy and security concerns surrounding the collection and storage of personal health information are critical issues that need to be addressed to ensure the trust and confidence of users. Additionally, bridging the digital divide and ensuring equal access to internet-based health platforms is crucial to prevent further disparities in healthcare.

In conclusion, the internet has the potential to revolutionize healthcare systems, making them more accessible, efficient, and patient-centric. From democratizing health information to enabling telemedicine and fostering the development of innovative healthcare technologies, the internet is reshaping the way we approach healthcare. However, it is important to address the challenges that come with it and ensure equal access to internet-based health platforms for all individuals. By embracing the digital wellness revolution, we can maximize the potential of the internet to improve healthcare outcomes for everyone.

In today's digital age, the internet has revolutionized almost every aspect of our lives, including the way we approach healthcare. With the rise of internet-based health platforms, there is a tremendous potential to transform healthcare systems worldwide. This subchapter explores the potential impact of these platforms on healthcare systems and how they can benefit all individuals in the internet niche.

Internet-based health platforms have the power to provide accessible and convenient healthcare services to everyone. With just a few clicks, individuals can connect with healthcare professionals, access medical information, and even receive virtual consultations. This accessibility breaks down traditional barriers to healthcare, allowing individuals in remote areas or those with limited mobility to receive the care they need.

Moreover, these platforms enable healthcare providers to deliver personalized care and improve patient outcomes. Through the collection and analysis of vast amounts of health data, providers can gain valuable insights into individual health profiles, facilitating more accurate diagnoses and treatment plans. This data-driven approach has the potential to revolutionize preventive care, allowing for early intervention and reducing the burden on healthcare systems.

Internet-based health platforms also foster patient empowerment and engagement. With the ability to access their health records, track their progress, and communicate with healthcare professionals, individuals can take an active role in managing their health. This increased engagement leads to better adherence to treatment plans, improved self-care, and ultimately, better health outcomes.

Furthermore, these platforms promote collaboration and knowledge sharing among healthcare professionals. Through secure networks, doctors, nurses, and specialists can collaborate, share expertise, and seek second opinions. This collective intelligence enhances the quality of care provided, leading to improved patient safety and better healthcare outcomes.

However, it is essential to address the challenges and concerns that come with the digital transformation of healthcare systems. Issues such as privacy, data security, and the digital divide must be carefully considered and addressed to ensure equitable access and protect patient information.

In conclusion, the potential impact of internet-based health platforms on healthcare systems is immense. From increasing accessibility to personalized care, promoting patient engagement, and fostering collaboration among healthcare professionals, these platforms have the power to revolutionize healthcare delivery. By embracing the digital wellness revolution, individuals in the internet niche can benefit from improved healthcare services that cater to their unique needs, ultimately leading to better health outcomes for everyone.

In today's digital age, the internet has revolutionized various aspects of our lives, and the healthcare system is no exception. The potential impact of internet-based health platforms on healthcare systems is one that cannot be ignored. This subchapter will explore the profound changes these platforms can bring and the benefits they offer to both individuals and healthcare providers.

Internet-based health platforms have the power to enhance the accessibility and convenience of healthcare services. With just a few clicks, individuals can access a wealth of health information, schedule appointments, and even seek remote consultations. This ease of access eliminates the need for physical visits to healthcare facilities, reducing the burden on traditional healthcare systems. For individuals in remote or underserved areas, internet-based platforms can bridge the gap by connecting them to healthcare professionals without the need for long-distance travel.

Furthermore, these platforms enable individuals to take control of their own health and well-being. With the availability of personalized health tracking tools, individuals can monitor their vital signs, track their exercise routines, and manage their diet. This empowers individuals to make proactive decisions regarding their health, leading to better self-management and prevention of chronic illnesses.

For healthcare providers, internet-based health platforms open up new avenues for patient care. Telemedicine, for instance, allows healthcare professionals to remotely diagnose and treat patients, increasing their reach and efficiency. This has proven especially beneficial during emergencies or when physical visits are not feasible, such as during a pandemic. Furthermore, these platforms enable healthcare providers to offer continuous care through remote monitoring of patients' health conditions, reducing hospital readmissions and improving overall healthcare outcomes.

However, it is important to address the challenges that may arise with the integration of internet-based health platforms into healthcare systems. Issues such as data security, privacy, and the digital divide must be carefully considered. Ensuring secure data transmission and storage, protecting patient privacy, and bridging the gap for individuals who lack access to the internet are crucial steps in maximizing the potential impact of these platforms.

In conclusion, the potential impact of internet-based health platforms on healthcare systems is immense. From enhancing accessibility and convenience to empowering individuals and transforming the way healthcare providers deliver care, these platforms have the potential to revolutionize the healthcare landscape. However, it is crucial to address the challenges and ensure a seamless integration of these platforms into healthcare systems, to truly maximize the benefits they offer to individuals and the healthcare industry as a whole.

Integrating Internet-based Health Platforms into Traditional Healthcare

In today's fast-paced digital era, the internet has revolutionized almost every aspect of our lives, including healthcare. With the rise of internet-based health platforms, individuals now have access to a vast array of resources and tools that can help them take control of their well-being. This subchapter explores the integration of these platforms into traditional healthcare systems, highlighting the benefits and challenges they pose for both healthcare providers and patients.

One of the primary advantages of integrating internet-based health platforms into traditional healthcare is the accessibility they offer. The internet has made it possible for individuals to access health-related information and services anytime, anywhere. Whether it's searching for symptoms, finding reputable health websites, or connecting with healthcare professionals through telemedicine, the internet has significantly expanded the reach of healthcare beyond the confines of physical clinics.

Moreover, internet-based health platforms empower individuals to actively participate in their own healthcare. Patients can now monitor their vitals, track their exercise routines, and even receive personalized health recommendations through various apps and wearable devices. This not only improves patient engagement but also enables healthcare professionals to gather more accurate and real-time data, leading to more precise diagnoses and personalized treatment plans.

However, integrating internet-based health platforms into traditional healthcare also presents several challenges. One of the most critical concerns is ensuring the security and privacy of patient data. As more sensitive health information is shared online, it becomes crucial for healthcare providers and platform developers to implement robust cybersecurity measures to protect patient confidentiality.

Additionally, bridging the gap between traditional healthcare and internet-based platforms requires effective collaboration and communication among healthcare providers, technology developers, and patients. Healthcare professionals need to be trained and educated on how to navigate and utilize these platforms effectively. Patients, on the other hand, need to be educated about the benefits and limitations of internet-based health platforms to make informed decisions regarding their own health.

In conclusion, integrating internet-based health platforms into traditional healthcare has the potential to revolutionize the way we approach and manage our well-being. However, it requires a careful balance between accessibility, security, and effective collaboration among all stakeholders involved. By harnessing the power of the internet, we can maximize the benefits of these platforms and empower individuals to take control of their health like never before. The digital wellness revolution is here, and it's time for everyone to embrace it.

In today's fast-paced digital world, the internet has become an integral part of our daily lives. It has revolutionized almost every aspect of our society, including healthcare. With the rise of internet-based health platforms, individuals now have access to a wealth of information, tools, and resources to manage their health and wellness effectively.

Internet-based health platforms encompass a wide range of digital tools and services that aim to improve healthcare outcomes and empower individuals to take control of their well-being. These platforms offer various functionalities such as health monitoring, symptom checkers, telemedicine services, online consultations, personalized health plans, and lifestyle management tools.

The integration of internet-based health platforms into traditional healthcare systems has immense potential to transform the way healthcare is delivered. It enables healthcare providers to extend their reach beyond physical clinics and hospitals, allowing them to connect with patients remotely and provide timely and convenient care. This integration also fosters patient engagement and encourages individuals to take an active role in managing their health.

For individuals, internet-based health platforms offer unparalleled convenience and accessibility. They can access their health records, track their progress, and communicate with healthcare providers at their convenience, eliminating the need for in-person appointments for routine healthcare needs. Patients can also gain valuable insights into their health status and receive personalized recommendations to improve their well-being.

Moreover, internet-based health platforms have a significant impact on preventive healthcare. They enable individuals to access information about healthy lifestyles, preventive measures, and early detection of diseases. This empowers people to make informed decisions about their health, leading to better health outcomes and reduced healthcare costs in the long run.

However, it is important to note that the integration of internet-based health platforms into traditional healthcare is not without challenges. Issues such as data privacy and security, regulatory compliance, and the digital divide need to be addressed to ensure the widespread adoption and effective implementation of these platforms.

In conclusion, integrating internet-based health platforms into traditional healthcare has the potential to revolutionize the healthcare industry. It empowers individuals to take control of their health and provides them with convenient access to healthcare services. By leveraging the power of the internet, we can maximize the potential of these platforms to improve health outcomes and promote a healthier society for everyone.

In today's digital era, the internet has revolutionized various aspects of our lives, and healthcare is no exception. The emergence of internet-based health platforms has paved the way for a new era of patient-centered care and has the potential to transform how we approach traditional healthcare practices. This subchapter explores the integration of internet-based health platforms into the traditional healthcare system, highlighting the benefits and challenges it brings for both patients and healthcare providers.

Internet-based health platforms offer numerous advantages, especially for individuals who are tech-savvy and have access to the internet. These platforms provide a wealth of information at our fingertips, allowing us to research medical conditions, access health records, and even consult with healthcare professionals through virtual visits. This increased accessibility and convenience save time and money for patients while reducing the burden on healthcare facilities.

For healthcare providers, integrating internet-based health platforms into traditional healthcare opens up opportunities for improved patient engagement and personalized care. These platforms enable healthcare professionals to monitor patients remotely, track their health progress, and provide timely interventions. Additionally, the integration of internet-based health platforms can streamline administrative tasks, such as appointment scheduling and prescription refills, allowing healthcare providers to focus more on patient care.

However, the integration of internet-based health platforms into traditional healthcare does not come without challenges. One major concern is the digital divide, as not everyone has equal access to the internet or possesses the necessary digital literacy skills. This discrepancy can exacerbate health inequalities and leave certain populations behind. Efforts must be made to bridge this gap and ensure that internet-based health platforms are accessible to everyone.

Another challenge is the potential for information overload and misinformation. With vast amounts of health information available online, it can be overwhelming for individuals to discern accurate and reliable sources. Healthcare providers play a crucial role in guiding patients towards trustworthy platforms and helping them navigate the digital landscape safely.

In conclusion, the integration of internet-based health platforms into traditional healthcare has the potential to revolutionize the way we approach healthcare. By leveraging the power of the internet, patients can access information, communicate with healthcare professionals, and actively participate in their own care. Healthcare providers can utilize these platforms to enhance patient engagement and deliver personalized care. However, it is essential to address challenges such as the digital divide and information overload to ensure that these platforms benefit everyone. The integration of internet-based health platforms is a significant step towards a more patient-centered and efficient healthcare system.

Redefining Healthcare Delivery Models

In today's digital era, the healthcare industry is undergoing a significant transformation. The advent of the internet has revolutionized the way healthcare services are delivered, paving the way for a new era of healthcare delivery models. This subchapter explores the various ways in which the internet has redefined healthcare delivery models and its impact on individuals across all walks of life.

The internet has opened up a world of possibilities when it comes to accessing healthcare services. With just a few clicks, individuals can now connect with healthcare providers, access medical information, and even receive consultations from the comfort of their own homes. This has resulted in a more convenient and accessible healthcare experience for everyone, regardless of their geographical location or personal circumstances.

One of the key ways in which the internet has redefined healthcare delivery models is through telemedicine. Telemedicine allows patients to connect with healthcare professionals remotely, eliminating the need for in-person visits and reducing the burden on healthcare facilities. This has been particularly beneficial for individuals living in remote areas or those with limited mobility, as it allows them to receive the care they need without the hassle of traveling long distances.

Furthermore, the internet has also given rise to a plethora of health and wellness platforms, catering to a wide range of niches. These platforms provide individuals with personalized health information, fitness programs, and even mental health support. The internet has democratized access to healthcare information, empowering individuals to take ownership of their own well-being.

In addition to telemedicine and wellness platforms, the internet has also facilitated the sharing of medical data and electronic health records. This has resulted in improved coordination of care, as healthcare providers can easily access and exchange patient information, leading to more accurate diagnoses and better treatment outcomes.

However, it is important to note that with the rise of the internet and digital health platforms, there are also challenges to consider. Privacy and security concerns surrounding the sharing of personal health information online need to be addressed to ensure the trust and confidence of individuals using these platforms.

In conclusion, the internet has revolutionized healthcare delivery models, making healthcare more accessible, convenient, and personalized for everyone. Telemedicine, wellness platforms, and the sharing of medical data have transformed the way healthcare is delivered, empowering individuals to take control of their own health. However, it is crucial to prioritize privacy and security to ensure the responsible use of digital health platforms. The future of healthcare lies in leveraging the power of the internet to create a truly patient-centered and efficient healthcare system.

In today's digital age, the internet has revolutionized various aspects of our lives, and healthcare is no exception. The emergence of internet-based health platforms has opened up new possibilities for accessing healthcare services, transforming the way we receive medical care. This subchapter explores the concept of redefining healthcare delivery models through the lens of the digital wellness revolution.

Internet-based health platforms have made healthcare more accessible and convenient for everyone. With just a few clicks, individuals can now connect with healthcare professionals, seek medical advice, and even receive diagnoses without leaving the comfort of their homes. This accessibility is particularly crucial for those who live in remote areas or have limited mobility, as it eliminates the barriers of distance and physical limitations.

These platforms also offer personalized healthcare experiences. By leveraging the power of data analytics and artificial intelligence, internet-based health platforms can analyze user data and provide tailored recommendations and treatments. This personalized approach not only enhances the overall quality of care but also empowers individuals to take charge of their own health and well-being.

Furthermore, internet-based health platforms have enabled the shift from a reactive to a proactive healthcare model. Instead of waiting for symptoms to manifest, individuals can now monitor their health in real-time through wearable devices and smartphone applications. These devices can track vital signs, sleep patterns, and physical activity, providing valuable insights into one's overall well-being. Armed with this information, individuals can make informed decisions about their lifestyle and seek preventive measures to maintain good health.

The digital wellness revolution has also facilitated better collaboration between healthcare providers and patients. Internet-based platforms allow for seamless communication and information sharing, enabling healthcare professionals to monitor patients remotely, provide timely advice, and even coordinate care with other specialists. This collaboration enhances the continuity of care and ensures that patients receive the best possible treatment.

In conclusion, the redefinition of healthcare delivery models through internet-based health platforms has transformed the way we access and receive healthcare services. These platforms offer accessibility, personalization, proactive care, and improved collaboration between healthcare providers and patients. The digital wellness revolution has the potential to empower individuals to take control of their health and lead healthier, more fulfilling lives. As the internet continues to evolve, so too will healthcare delivery models, ultimately benefiting everyone in the pursuit of better health.

Chapter 7: Conclusion

Recap of Key Takeaways

In this subchapter, we will summarize the key takeaways from the book "The Digital Wellness Revolution: Maximizing Internet-based Health Platforms." These takeaways will be beneficial to everyone, regardless of their level of familiarity with the internet and its various niches.

1. The Power of Internet-based Health Platforms: The internet has brought about a revolution in the field of healthcare by providing easily accessible platforms for individuals to monitor and manage their well-being. These platforms offer a wide range of services, including health tracking, telemedicine, online support groups, and personalized health recommendations.

2. Embracing Digital Wellness: Digital wellness refers to using internet-based tools and platforms to enhance one's overall well-being. It involves being mindful of our digital habits, setting boundaries, and utilizing technology to support our physical and mental health goals. By embracing digital wellness, we can harness the power of the internet to improve our lives.

3. Health Tracking and Monitoring: Internet-based health platforms allow individuals to track and monitor various aspects of their health, such as physical activity, sleep patterns, heart rate, and nutrition. These tools provide valuable insights into our daily habits and enable us to make informed decisions about our health.

4. Telemedicine and Virtual Consultations: The internet has made healthcare more accessible through telemedicine and virtual consultations. These services allow individuals to consult with healthcare professionals remotely, saving time and eliminating geographical barriers. Telemedicine has particularly proved beneficial during the COVID-19 pandemic, ensuring continuity of care while minimizing the risk of infection.

5. Online Support Communities: The internet has transformed the way people seek support and connect with others facing similar health challenges. Online support communities provide a safe space for individuals to share their experiences, seek advice, and find emotional support. These communities can be particularly helpful for individuals with rare diseases or conditions, who may not have access to local support groups.

6. Personalized Health Recommendations: Internet-based health platforms leverage data analytics and artificial intelligence to provide personalized health recommendations. By analyzing an individual's health data, these platforms can offer tailored advice, such as exercise routines, dietary suggestions, and stress management techniques. This personalized approach to healthcare empowers individuals to take control of their well-being.

In conclusion, the internet has revolutionized the field of healthcare, offering individuals a wealth of opportunities to improve their well-being. By embracing digital wellness, utilizing health tracking tools, embracing telemedicine, joining online support communities, and benefiting from personalized health recommendations, we can harness the power of the internet to maximize our health and wellness.

Whether you are an internet enthusiast or someone new to the digital world, these key takeaways will help you navigate and leverage the internet-based health platforms available to you.

In this fast-paced digital era, the internet has revolutionized various aspects of our lives, including the way we manage our health and wellness. "The Digital Wellness Revolution: Maximizing Internet-based Health Platforms" is a comprehensive guidebook that explores the potential of internet-based health platforms and the impact they can have on our well-being. As we conclude this enlightening journey, let's recap some of the key takeaways that can benefit everyone, especially those interested in the internet and its niches.

1. Empowerment through Information: The internet provides an abundance of health-related information at our fingertips. However, it is crucial to verify the credibility of sources and consult professionals for accurate advice. Use internet-based health platforms as tools to educate yourself and make informed decisions about your well-being.

2. Personalized Health Management: Internet-based health platforms offer personalized solutions that cater to individual needs. By utilizing these platforms, you can track your progress, set goals, and receive tailored recommendations. Embrace the power of technology to enhance your overall health.

3. Telemedicine and Remote Care: The internet has brought healthcare directly to our homes. Telemedicine allows individuals to consult healthcare professionals remotely, saving time and cost. Embrace virtual doctor visits, online therapy, and remote monitoring for a convenient and efficient healthcare experience.

4. Mental Health and Digital Detox: The constant exposure to screens and digital devices can negatively impact our mental health. Practice digital detox by setting boundaries, limiting screen time, and engaging in activities that promote mindfulness and relaxation. Prioritize mental well-being in this digital age.

5. Online Support Communities: The internet connects like-minded individuals and creates communities focused on specific health concerns. Engage in online support groups to share experiences, gain insights, and find emotional support. Collaborate with others who understand your journey and can provide guidance.

6. Data Privacy and Security: As we embrace internet-based health platforms, it is essential to prioritize data privacy and security. Be cautious while sharing personal information and ensure that the platforms you use adhere to strict privacy policies.

7. Continuous Learning and Adaptation: The digital wellness revolution is an ever-evolving landscape. Stay updated with the latest technological advancements, research, and best practices. Embrace a growth mindset, be open to new ideas, and adapt to changes as they occur.

Remember, the internet is a powerful tool that can improve our health and well-being if used responsibly. Embrace the digital wellness revolution, maximize internet-based health platforms, and take charge of your overall well-being in this digital age.

As we come to the end of this book, "The Digital Wellness Revolution: Maximizing Internet-based Health Platforms," it's important to recap the key takeaways that will empower each and every one of us to navigate the vast world of the internet and its impact on our health and well-being.

In today's digital age, the internet plays a significant role in our lives, particularly in relation to our health. With the rise of internet-based health platforms, it has become easier than ever to access information, connect with healthcare professionals, and track our own wellness journey. However, it is crucial to approach this digital wellness revolution with caution and mindfulness.

First and foremost, we must prioritize our digital well-being. While the internet provides a wealth of information, it is equally important to unplug, disconnect, and find balance in our lives. Setting boundaries and establishing healthy technology habits can help us maintain a healthy relationship with the digital world.

Secondly, understanding the credibility and reliability of internet-based health platforms is paramount. With the abundance of information available online, it's crucial to critically evaluate sources, fact-check claims, and consult professionals when necessary. Being discerning consumers of online health information can help us make informed decisions about our well-being.

Additionally, the book highlights the importance of privacy and security in the digital realm. With our personal health data being stored and shared online, it is essential to take steps to protect our privacy and ensure the security of our information. Being aware of the privacy policies of the platforms we use, using strong passwords, and being cautious about sharing personal information are some of the key strategies discussed.

Moreover, the book emphasizes the power of community and connection in the digital wellness revolution. Engaging with online support groups, seeking virtual healthcare communities, and utilizing social media platforms mindfully can foster a sense of belonging and provide valuable support in our health journeys.

Lastly, the book encourages us to embrace the opportunities that internet-based health platforms offer. From telemedicine and virtual consultations to apps that track our fitness and nutrition, these platforms have the potential to revolutionize healthcare and empower individuals to take control of their well-being.

In conclusion, "The Digital Wellness Revolution: Maximizing Internet-based Health Platforms" serves as a guide for every individual navigating the internet and its impact on their health. By prioritizing digital well-being, critically evaluating information, protecting our privacy, embracing community, and utilizing digital health platforms wisely, we can maximize the benefits of the internet while safeguarding our overall well-being.

Embracing the Digital Wellness Revolution

In today's fast-paced world, the internet has become an integral part of our lives. From social media platforms to online shopping and virtual communication, the internet has revolutionized the way we interact and access information. However, with its numerous benefits, the digital age also brings with it several challenges to our well-being. The concept of digital wellness has emerged as a response to these challenges, aiming to maximize the positive impact of internet-based health platforms while minimizing their potential negative effects.

Digital wellness encompasses a wide range of practices and strategies that promote a healthy and balanced relationship with technology. It encourages individuals to be mindful of their digital usage and to harness the power of the internet for their well-being. By embracing the digital wellness revolution, we can tap into the immense potential of the internet while effectively managing its impact on our mental, emotional, and physical health.

One of the key aspects of digital wellness is cultivating a healthy digital diet. Just as we carefully choose and monitor our food intake, we should be mindful of the content we consume online. This involves being aware of the time we spend on social media, news websites, and other online platforms, as well as the type of content we engage with. By curating our digital diet, we can ensure that we are exposed to positive, informative, and inspiring content that enhances our well-being.

Another essential component of digital wellness is establishing healthy boundaries with technology. It is crucial to set limits on screen time and create designated "tech-free" zones or periods in our daily lives. By creating space for offline activities, such as exercise, hobbies, and face-to-face interactions, we can maintain a healthy balance between our virtual and real-world experiences.

Furthermore, the digital wellness revolution encourages the use of internet-based health platforms to enhance our overall well-being. From fitness apps and online therapy sessions to mindfulness meditation programs and nutrition trackers, the internet offers a plethora of tools and resources to support our health goals. By leveraging these platforms, we can access valuable information, connect with like-minded individuals, and receive personalized support, all from the comfort of our own homes.

In conclusion, embracing the digital wellness revolution is essential for individuals in the internet age. By adopting a mindful approach to technology, curating our digital consumption, and utilizing internet-based health platforms, we can harness the power of the internet to optimize our well-being. Through this revolution, we can find balance, connection, and empowerment in the digital world, ultimately leading healthier and happier lives.

In today's fast-paced, interconnected world, the internet has become an integral part of our lives. From social media to online shopping, we rely on the internet for various aspects of our daily routines. However, the internet's impact on our well-being has been a topic of concern in recent years. This subchapter aims to shed light on the digital wellness revolution and how embracing it can positively transform our lives.

The digital wellness revolution refers to the growing movement towards maximizing internet-based health platforms to improve our overall well-being. These platforms offer a plethora of resources and tools designed to help individuals take charge of their physical, mental, and emotional health. From fitness apps and meditation guides to online therapy sessions and virtual support groups, the digital wellness revolution provides endless possibilities for self-care and personal growth.

One of the key benefits of embracing the digital wellness revolution is the convenience it offers. With a few clicks, we can access a wide range of health-related services, eliminating the need for physical appointments or travel. This accessibility empowers individuals from all walks of life to prioritize their well-being, regardless of their geographical location or time constraints.

Moreover, the internet's vast reach allows for the democratization of health information. Internet-based health platforms provide valuable educational resources, making it easier for individuals to understand and manage their health conditions. Whether it's learning about proper nutrition, tracking exercise routines, or seeking advice from medical professionals, the internet enables us to become active participants in our own health journeys.

Furthermore, the digital wellness revolution has the potential to foster a sense of community and support. Through online forums and social media groups, individuals can connect with like-minded individuals who share similar health goals or challenges. This virtual support system can provide encouragement, motivation, and a safe space for individuals to share their experiences and seek guidance.

However, it is essential to approach the digital wellness revolution mindfully. While the internet offers incredible resources, it is crucial to strike a balance and avoid excessive screen time or over-reliance on digital platforms. Setting boundaries, being aware of potential privacy concerns, and seeking credible sources are critical aspects of embracing the digital wellness revolution responsibly.

In conclusion, the digital wellness revolution presents a tremendous opportunity for individuals to take control of their health and well-being. By embracing internet-based health platforms, we can access a plethora of resources, improve convenience, and foster a sense of community. However, it is crucial to approach this revolution with mindfulness and responsibility. Ultimately, by harnessing the power of the internet, we can maximize our potential for personal growth and lead healthier, more fulfilling lives.

In today's fast-paced world, where the internet plays an integral role in our daily lives, it has become crucial to prioritize our digital wellness. The digital revolution has brought unparalleled convenience and connectivity, but it has also presented new challenges to our overall well-being. In this subchapter, we will explore the importance of embracing the digital wellness revolution and maximizing internet-based health platforms.

The internet has revolutionized the way we access information and connect with others. From social media platforms to health-tracking apps, the online world offers a vast array of resources to improve our well-being. However, it is also easy to get overwhelmed or consumed by the constant flow of information, leading to issues such as digital burnout or excessive screen time. By embracing the digital wellness revolution, we can harness the power of the internet while safeguarding our mental, emotional, and physical health.

One of the key aspects of the digital wellness revolution is becoming intentional with our online activities. It is crucial to set boundaries and find a healthy balance between our digital and offline lives. By prioritizing self-care and practicing mindful internet use, we can reap the benefits of technology without falling victim to its downsides. This subchapter will provide practical tips and strategies for creating a digital wellness plan that works for you.

Furthermore, we will delve into the various internet-based health platforms available. These platforms offer a wide range of services, from virtual doctor visits to mental health support. The convenience of accessing healthcare remotely has become particularly clear during the global pandemic, making internet-based health platforms an essential tool in our modern world. We will explore how these platforms can empower individuals to take charge of their health, providing access to information, resources, and professional support at their fingertips.

Regardless of our age or background, the internet has become an integral part of our lives. Embracing the digital wellness revolution is not about rejecting technology but rather about using it mindfully and purposefully. By understanding the potential risks and rewards of the online world, we can navigate it safely and reap its many benefits.

In conclusion, this subchapter aims to inspire and empower readers to embrace the digital wellness revolution. It will provide practical guidance on setting boundaries, practicing mindfulness, and maximizing the potential of internet-based health platforms. By taking control of our digital well-being, we can lead healthier, more balanced lives in this increasingly connected world.

Empowering Individuals through Internet-based Health Platforms

In today's digital age, the internet has revolutionized every aspect of our lives, including how we approach our health and well-being. Internet-based health platforms have emerged as powerful tools that empower individuals to take control of their own health. This subchapter explores how these platforms are transforming the way we access healthcare information, connect with healthcare professionals, and manage our personal health.

The internet has opened up a world of possibilities when it comes to accessing healthcare information. With just a few clicks, individuals can now find a wealth of knowledge on various health topics, from symptoms and treatments to preventive measures and lifestyle changes. Internet-based health platforms provide a vast array of resources, such as articles, videos, and infographics, that enable individuals to educate themselves and make informed decisions about their health.

Additionally, these platforms have facilitated the connection between individuals and healthcare professionals. Online consultations, telemedicine, and virtual health services have become increasingly popular, allowing individuals to seek medical advice and treatment from the comfort of their homes. This is particularly beneficial for those living in remote areas or with limited mobility, as it eliminates geographical barriers and improves access to healthcare services.

Internet-based health platforms also play a crucial role in empowering individuals to manage their personal health. Through the use of innovative tools and trackers, individuals can monitor their vital signs, track their physical activity, and even manage chronic conditions. These platforms provide personalized insights and recommendations, helping individuals make positive lifestyle changes and maintain a healthy lifestyle.

Furthermore, internet-based health platforms foster a sense of community and support. Online forums, support groups, and social media communities bring together individuals facing similar health challenges, creating a space for sharing experiences, seeking advice, and providing emotional support. This online connectivity helps individuals feel less alone in their health journeys and encourages them to actively participate in their own well-being.

While internet-based health platforms offer numerous advantages, it is essential for individuals to use them responsibly and critically evaluate the information they find online. It is always recommended to consult with healthcare professionals for accurate diagnosis and personalized advice.

In conclusion, the advent of internet-based health platforms has revolutionized the way individuals approach their health. These platforms empower individuals to access healthcare information, connect with healthcare professionals, manage their personal health, and find support within online communities. By harnessing the power of the internet, individuals can take control of their well-being, leading to a healthier, more informed society.

In today's digital era, the internet has become an indispensable tool in our everyday lives. It has revolutionized the way we communicate, work, and access information. However, one of the most significant advancements brought about by the internet is its impact on healthcare. Internet-based health platforms have emerged as powerful tools that empower individuals to take control of their well-being and make informed decisions about their health.

The internet has made healthcare accessible to everyone, regardless of their geographic location or socio-economic background. Internet-based health platforms provide a wealth of information on various health conditions, preventive measures, and treatment options. From trusted medical websites to online forums and support groups, individuals can now access a vast knowledge base at their fingertips. This democratization of health information ensures that everyone has equal access to valuable resources, enabling them to make informed decisions about their health.

Moreover, internet-based health platforms offer a range of tools and services that empower individuals to actively monitor and manage their health. From fitness trackers and wearable devices to mobile apps and telemedicine services, these platforms provide individuals with real-time health data and personalized recommendations. This enables individuals to track their progress, set goals, and make necessary adjustments in their lifestyle to improve their overall well-being.

For individuals with chronic conditions, internet-based health platforms offer a lifeline of support and guidance. Online communities and forums provide a safe space for individuals to connect, share experiences, and seek advice from others facing similar challenges. This sense of community and support can be invaluable in managing chronic conditions and can significantly improve an individual's quality of life.

Internet-based health platforms also play a crucial role in preventive healthcare. With the rise of telemedicine and virtual consultations, individuals can now access healthcare professionals from the comfort of their own homes. This not only saves time and money but also encourages proactive healthcare-seeking behaviors. Regular check-ups, early detection of diseases, and timely interventions can prevent the progression of conditions and improve long-term health outcomes.

In conclusion, internet-based health platforms have revolutionized the way individuals access and manage their healthcare. By providing equal access to information, personalized tools, and support networks, these platforms empower individuals to take charge of their well-being. The internet has truly transformed healthcare, making it more accessible, inclusive, and individual-centric. As we embrace the digital wellness revolution, it is crucial for everyone to harness the power of internet-based health platforms to maximize their health potential.

In today's digital age, the internet has become an integral part of our lives, revolutionizing the way we communicate, work, and even take care of our health. Internet-based health platforms have emerged as powerful tools that empower individuals to take control of their well-being, offering a wealth of information, resources, and support at their fingertips. This subchapter explores the immense potential of internet-based health platforms in transforming the way we approach and manage our health.

The internet has democratized access to health information, enabling individuals from all walks of life to educate themselves about various health conditions, preventive measures, and treatment options.

Internet-based health platforms offer a vast repository of reliable and up-to-date information that can be accessed anytime, anywhere, and by anyone with an internet connection. Whether you are looking for dietary advice, exercise routines, or information about a specific medical condition, these platforms provide a wealth of resources to aid in making informed decisions about your health.

Moreover, internet-based health platforms foster a sense of community and support among individuals with similar health concerns. Online forums, support groups, and social media platforms dedicated to health-related topics allow individuals to connect, share experiences, and provide emotional support to one another. This virtual support system can be especially beneficial for those facing rare or stigmatized health conditions, who may find it challenging to find support in their immediate surroundings.

Internet-based health platforms also enable individuals to actively participate in their own healthcare journey. Through features like telemedicine, remote monitoring, and health tracking apps, individuals can easily communicate with healthcare professionals, monitor their health parameters, and access personalized care plans from the comfort of their homes. This not only improves convenience but also enhances the overall quality of care, ensuring that individuals have timely access to the resources they need to manage their health effectively.

However, it is essential to recognize the potential challenges and limitations of internet-based health platforms. The vast amount of information available online can be overwhelming, and not all sources may be trustworthy or credible. It is crucial for individuals to exercise critical thinking and consult healthcare professionals before making any major decisions regarding their health. Additionally, the digital divide and disparities in internet access and technological literacy can hinder the full potential of these platforms, preventing some individuals from benefiting from the transformative power of internet-based health resources.

In conclusion, internet-based health platforms have revolutionized the way we approach our health by empowering individuals with information, resources, and support. By leveraging the power of the internet, individuals can now take an active role in managing their well-being, connecting with others, and accessing personalized care. As the digital wellness revolution continues to unfold, it is crucial to ensure equal access and promote digital literacy to maximize the benefits of internet-based health platforms for everyone.

www.ingramcontent.com/pod-product-compliance
Lightning Source LLC
LaVergne TN
LVHW021825060526
838201LV00058B/3517